Successful Transition
to Practice

Successful Transition to Practice

A GUIDE FOR THE NEW NURSE PRACTITIONER

**Deborah L. Dillon, DNP, RN, ACNP-BC,
CCRN, CHFN-K**
Associate Professor and Director of the AGACNP Program
School of Nursing
Duquesne University
Pittsburgh, Pennsylvania

New York   Chicago   San Francisco   Athens
London   Madrid   Mexico City   Milan
New Delhi   Singapore   Sydney   Toronto

3360   KH

Successful Transition to Practice: A Guide for the New Nurse Practitioner

1 2 3 4 5 6 7 8 9   LCR   26 25 24 23 22 21

ISBN 978-1-260-45237-2
MHID 1-260-45237-9

This book was set in Minion Pro by MPS Limited.
The editors were Susan Oldenburg and Peter J. Boyle.
The production supervisor was Richard Ruzycka.
The text was designed by Eve Siegel.
The cover designer was W2 Design.
Project management was provided by Touseen Qadri, MPS Limited.

This book is printed on acid-free paper.

Cataloging-in-Publication data for this book is on file at the Library of Congress.

McGraw Hill books are available at special quantity discounts to use as premiums and sales promotions or for use in corporate training programs. To contact a representative, please visit the Contact Us pages at www.mhprofessional.com.

8/16/21

CONTENTS

FOREWORD

Lead. Practice. Transform. These words apply to the vision, endorsed by the American Association of Colleges of Nursing (AACN) in 2004, that the entry level for all advanced practice nurses should be the DNP degree. Though the 2015 target date for full implementation of that vision has passed, the vision is still clear that the complexity of the U.S. healthcare system demands that advanced practice nurses (APRNs) practice at the highest level of education and to the full scope of their education, certification, and licensure. While education is essential, transition to practice is equally important. Any transition to a new role comes with both rewards and challenges. Dr. Deborah Dillon, associate professor and director of the AGACNP program at Duquesne University School of Nursing and a practicing acute care nurse practitioner, helps APRNs to meet this challenge by providing this critical text.

Lead. The chapters in this text, as edited by Dr. Dillon, provide the building blocks for the APRN to take a leadership role in applying evidence-based care to patients and populations. Such leadership starts with a commitment to consumer safety as recognized by national certification so nicely detailed in Chapter 2 on national certification.

Practice. The DNP is considered to be the practice doctorate and highlights the core precept of advanced practice nursing— that it is through doing, caring, and reasoning that the APRN produces outcomes for patient and their families and the systems that deliver this care. However, the advanced practice role has many complex layers that are made less complex by several chapters in this text including those on state licensure, full practice authority, and fellowships.

Transform. Change is needed in the U.S. healthcare system and the challenges facing providers, payers, and consumers are well documented. Doctorally prepared APRNs need a framework to optimize their transition into practice because the need is great and the time is now. Many chapters in Dr. Dillon's highly relevant text will help the APRN to transform—at the personal level and the practice level. Chapter 1 on the DNP degree and Chapters 6 and 7 on contracts and negotiating salary are pertinent to such transformation.

As a consumer of healthcare and an educator of future APRNs, I commend Dr. Dillon for this timely and essential text. Transition to practice for APRNs has been made clearer by this text. I hope that all APRN students and new APRNs will read this text in order to lead, practice, and transform.

Clareen Wiencek, PhD, RN, ACNP
Director of Advanced Practice
University of Virginia School of Nursing

Successful Transition to Practice

1 Planning for Graduation

Planning for graduation starts prior to enrollment in your nurse practitioner (NP) program. You your unique university as well as your specialty tract. These are the two big steps in this process. You had to do some research on what specific program met your educational needs. Do you prefer in class or on-line learning? What are the university's statistics regarding program completion, board certification, and availability of clinical placements? Are you obtaining a Masters in Nursing or Doctorate of Nursing Practice? Other factors such as proximity, class size, and cost probably played a role in your decision as well. You also have spent a great deal of self-reflection contemplating what area of practice you wanted to go into. None of these decisions are taken lightly. You have made a decision regarding your future nursing career.

Realistically, the true planning for graduation starts at the time you enroll in your NP program. Although graduation may not always be at the forefront of your daily thoughts, it should be with you as you progress through your academic program. By keeping your "eye on graduation" you will stay organized and keep track of various educational materials that will be required both at and after graduation. Copies of course syllabi and documentation of clinical hours and procedures are just a few of the items you will want to include in a database early on in your NP program. You may choose to store your data as hard copies, electronically, or both. Keeping this information in a designated area, such as using it to start your portfolio, is a great way for the initial organizing of this important data. There are several areas that will be great resources to guide your practice. They have already been utilized in shaping your NP program. These three areas are the Advanced Practice Registered Nurse (APRN) Consensus Model,[1] the National Organization of Nurse Practitioner Faculties (NONPF) competencies,[2] and the American Association of Colleges of Nursing's (AACN) NP Curriculum Guidelines and Core Competencies.[3]

APRN CONSENSUS MODEL

In 2008 the Consensus Model for APRN Regulation was released by the AACN. AACN and the National Council of State Boards of Nursing (NCSBN) facilitated the consensus building used to develop this model. One of the goals of the Consensus Model was to provide state-to-state uniformity in the regulation of APRN roles. As long as continued differences are allowed to occur between states, obstacles to license portability exist. The Consensus Model for APRNs is a document that describes the APRN regulatory model, identifies titles to be used, defines specialty, describes the emergence of new roles and population foci, and presents strategies for implementation.[1]

The Consensus Model for APRN Regulation defines advanced practice registered nurse practice and describes emergence of new roles and population foci.[1] Often referred to as LACE (licensure, accreditation, certification, and education), this model adopted the term "population focus" to describe the broad area of preparation for NPs. This landmark model defined titles to be used by NPs, defined emergence of new roles and specialty populations (or population foci), and presented strategies for implementation.[4] Your NP specialty track was developed based on the APRN Consensus Model. Details regarding your specific population focus can be found in this document.[1]

Over the past several decades the APRN has become a highly valued and integral part of the healthcare system. Hence, this is probably one of the reasons you have chosen this career pathway. APRNs include practitioners in the following four areas: (1) certified registered nurse anesthetists (CRNA), (2) certified nurse midwives (CNM), (3) clinical nurse specialists (CNS), and (4) certified nurse practitioners (CNP). While each of these APRN roles is unique in its history and development, they share the common characteristic of being an advanced practice role. The uniqueness of these individual practitioners is that their role focuses on specialized knowledge and skills acquired through graduate or doctoral-level education. These APRN roles focus on direct patient care.

The APRN Consensus Model focuses on these four, specific advanced practice roles. Registered nurses with advanced graduate education (e.g., education, management, public health) are not included in this model as their practice is for the advancement of the health of the public, not that of direct care to individuals. It is for this reason that their roles are not subject to the Regulatory Model that is addressed in the APRN Consensus Model.[1]

The APRN Consensus Model represents the four APRN roles—CRNA, CNM, CNS, and CNP as well as the six population foci. The population foci within the NP role include family/individual across lifespan, adult-gerontology, neonatal, pediatrics, women's health/gender related, and psychiatric/mental health. Within the pediatric and adult-gerontology population foci there is both a primary care and acute care preparation. Education, licensure, and certification must be congruent in terms of role and population foci.[1] APRN educational programs must be accredited by a nursing accreditation organization that is recognized by the U.S. Department of Education (USDE) and/or the Council for Higher Education Accreditation (CHEA). Examples are as follows:

- Commission on Collegiate Nursing Education (CCNE)
- National League for Nursing Accrediting Commission (NLNAC)
- Council on Accreditation of Nurse Anesthesia Educational Programs (COA)
- Accreditation Commission for Midwifery Education (ACME)
- National Association of Nurse Practitioners in Women's Health Council on Accreditation

After the APRN has completed the required education, he/she will sit for a national certification examination to assess competencies of the APRN core, role, and at least one defined population foci (i.e., adult-gerontology primary care). APRN certification programs are required to be accredited by a national certification accrediting body. The certification program should be nationally accredited by the American Board of Nursing Specialties (ABNS) or the National Commission for Certifying Agencies (NCCA). APRN certification programs require a continued competency mechanism.

The APRN Consensus Model is often referred to as LACE: licensure, accreditation, certification, and education. The formal definitions per the APRN Consensus Model are as follows:

- **Licensure** is referred to as the granting of authority to practice.
- **Accreditation** is the formal review and approval process by a recognized agency of an educational degree or certification program in nursing or nursing-related programs.
- **Certification** is the formal recognition of the knowledge, skills, and experience demonstrated by the achievement of standards identified by the profession.
- **Education** refers to the formal preparation of APRNs in graduate degree-granting or postgraduate certificate programs.

APRN ROLE DEFINED

An APRN is defined by the document as a nurse who has completed an accredited, graduate, postgraduate, or doctoral-level education program in one of the four recognized APRN roles. This individual has then passed a national certification examination recognized by a national certification program. This advanced practice nurse has acquired advanced clinical knowledge and skills preparing him/her to provide direct care to patients, as well as a component of indirect care. The main focus of practice is that of direct care of individuals. This nurse is educationally prepared to assume responsibility and accountability for health promotion and/or maintenance as well as assessment, diagnosis, and management of patient problems which include the use of pharmacologic and nonpharmacologic interventions. The advanced practice nurse also has clinical experience of sufficient depth and breadth to reflect the intended license, and has obtained a license to practice as an APRN in one of the four APRN roles.[1]

NATIONAL ORGANIZATION OF NURSE PRACTITIONER FACULTIES (NONPF)

NONPF, which was formed in 1976, was developed to support the development of instructional skills and scientific investigation in NP education. In its early years, NONPF focused on establishing curriculum guidelines for NP education. Its continued mission is to be the leader in quality NP education. Since 1990, NONPF has identified core competencies for all NPs.[2] These core competencies, with the most recent update being in 2017, represent all NPs' entry into practice competencies upon their graduation from an accredited NP program. NONPF's organizational goals are to promote excellence in NP education through creation of evidence-based strategies and resources in teaching, research, practice, and service. Finally, NONPF promotes engagement by leveraging the membership as a valuable resource to advance the mission and vision of its organization.[2]

Utilizing the population focus of the Consensus Model for APRN Regulation,[1] a multiorganizational task force completed the following competencies for various NP population foci. The implementation date is associated with its specific specialty.

- 2010 Adult-Gerontology Primary Care Nurse Practitioners
- 2012 Adult-Gerontology Acute Care Nurse Practitioners
- 2013 Primary Care Pediatric Nurse Practitioner
- 2013 Acute Care Pediatric Nurse Practitioner

- 2013 Neonatal Nurse Practitioner
- Family/Across the Lifespan Nurse Practitioner
- Women's Health/Gender-Related Nurse Practitioner
- Psychiatric/Mental Health

Although these competencies guide NP programs and add structure, there are still unique characteristics of each NP program nationally. NONPF has outlined competencies for each of these specialty population foci. The broad competency categories developed include scientific foundation, leadership, quality, practice inquiry, technology information and literacy, policy, health delivery system, ethics, and independent practice.

In 2006, NONPF introduced the Doctor of Nursing Practice (DNP) Nurse Practitioner Competencies. These competencies were built on the already existing core population-focused competencies for NPs. In 2011, these competencies were replaced by a single set of NP core competencies.[2] The 2017 NP Core Competencies with Suggested Curriculum Content were developed with suggested doctoral-level curriculum content to support the competencies.[2]

Both the APRN Consensus Model and the NONPF Competencies define the specific differences in the various NP specialty programs. Referring to these documents is an extremely helpful resource in understanding your scope of practice. At present, each state has its own Scope of Practice (SOP) which may further delineate or restrict your practice. You will want to familiarize yourself with all of these documents as you move through your NP program and refer to them frequently after graduation.

AMERICAN ASSOCIATION OF COLLEGES OF NURSING

AACN[3] has several areas that address NPs. The Master of Science in Nursing (MSN) 2011 and Doctoral Nursing Practice

(DNP) 2006 Essentials guide advanced practice nursing. These essentials also provide the framework for developing the MSN and DNP curricula. The essentials are used nationally by nursing deans and faculty to design curricula to prepare highly qualified nurses for a health system in continual change.[3] The essentials address the expected competencies of graduates from these specific nursing programs. In order for nursing education programs to be accredited by the CCNE, these competencies are core for all advanced nursing practice roles.[3] The essentials are available online and can be downloaded for free.

AACN also defines curriculum standards for the advanced practice roles. These guidelines provide a framework for "positioning graduate-degree nursing programs to meet the healthcare challenges of a new century." Below is a list of the specific competencies and their associated year of implementation.[3]

- Adult-Gerontology Primary Care Nurse Practitioner Competencies (2016)
- Adult-Gerontology Acute Care Nurse Practitioner Competencies (2012)
- Nurse Practitioner Core Competencies Content (2014)
- Population-focused Nurse Practitioner Competencies (2013)
- Psychiatric-Mental Health Nurse Practitioner Competencies (2014)

In 2017, AACN developed the APRN Doctoral-Level Competencies and Progression Indicators. The significance of this work is that it represents a first step in the transition to competency-based education. This work will hopefully move the transition from time-based education (NP requirement of a minimum of 500 clinical hours to sit for most board certification examinations) and clinical experiences to standardized, competency-based assessment which would mirror the process currently underway in other health professions (i.e., medicine).[3] There are eight domains. Within each domain there are various competency levels. For each level of competency there are two progression indicators—noted as Time 1 and Time 2. Time 1 "describes the expected level of achievement when the student begins the first meaningful clinical experience where the student provides direct patient care management under preceptor or faculty supervision." Time 2 "describes the expected level of performance at completion of the student's APRN doctoral program (graduation)."[3]

You may recognize one additional branch of the AACN—the CCNE. CCNE is the national accreditation agency, which is a part of the office of the AACN. They are a voluntary, self-regulatory agency that supports and encourages continuing self-assessment by nursing programs and supports continuing growth and improvement of collegiate professional education and nurse residency programs.[4] They are one of the organizations that accredits nursing programs.

Program Course Materials

Retaining course materials is essential. Program course content can vary significantly over time. It is a good idea to retain copies of all course syllabi organized by subject. Electronic copies from your program may allow you limited or no access after the course is completed or after graduation. Saving a hard copy or an electronic file is strongly recommended. This makes this data easily retrievable should you need it for future access. Courses are revised regularly as well, so what is being offered in the program today may not be identical to content from 2 years ago. You should start organizing these materials from day one of your program. Course syllabi are your documentation as to the objectives, course hours, overall course description, and specific content that was addressed in your program's curriculum. These syllabi may be requested for review by a future employer or hospital credentialing committee. The course information is also required by the national board certification agencies. Information regarding the course hours, course number, year

TABLE 1-1

Sample Course Log

Month/ Year taken	Course title	Course number	Course description	Credit hours
August– December 2018	Advanced Pathophysiology	GNUR 1234	See attached syllabus or may be cited from the original syllabus	4.0
January– May 2019	Advanced Pharmacology	GNUR 1245	See attached syllabus or may be cited from the original syllabus	4.0

taken, and credit hours is some of the data that is required (Table 1-1).

Course Sequencing

At this point in time, it is important to have a discussion on course sequencing. Most programs outline the sequencing for NP courses. The 3Ps—pharmacology, pathophysiology, and advanced health assessment, are often "front-loaded" in NP curriculum as they are foundational courses. Your curriculum building block is another way of looking at them. However, there is usually some degree of latitude in this approach. Course sequencing, particularly related to pharmacology, is often the course that can become problematic. Per NONPF recommendations, pharmacology should be taken prior to or concurrent with your first clinical practicum course.[2] There have been instances in which students took their pharmacology course very early in their program and then experienced unexpected delays in program completion (sometimes referred to as life events—illness, pregnancy, family issues are just a few examples). Individual states have their own requirements on the time frame from completion of your pharmacology course and initial licensure. Some states have a 3- or 5-year time requirement (i.e., Virginia). This time limitation has required students who fell into this category of "being out of sequence" to take an additional pharmacology course. Prior to enrolling in a pharmacology course, consult with your specific State Board of Nursing and program faculty for course approval. You will want to be sure the pharmacology course you select is acceptable to your State Board of Nursing and that you have their written approval that the course meets their requirements before you incur this additional time and expense.

Although there are commonalities between NP programs, there are also differences that may support your privileging requests (e.g., exposure to surgical technique). For example, your NP program may have had an emphasis in palliative care or you may have chosen this as an area of focus for one of your practicums. If this is an area where you will be seeking employment post graduation, it will be important that you can provide course descriptions, lecture content, and clinical hours related to the specialty area. The names and certifications of your preceptors are also significant data to include.

Clinical Hour Requirements

All NP programs have a clinical hour requirement. The clinical hours may vary from program to program and from specialty to specialty within the same programs. The specified clinical hour requirement depends upon your university program and may range from the minimum of 500 to 750 clinical hours. Clinical hour requirements vary based on the specific population focus and the individual nursing program. This means that within the same school/college of nursing there may be different time/clinical hour requirements depending on the NP population foci. For example, a Family Nurse Practitioner program may require a completion of 750 hours and the Adult Primary

Care Nurse Practitioner program may require the minimum of 500 clinical hours. The National Task Force (NTF) on Quality Nurse Practitioner Education recognizes that NP programs are moving to improve outcome assessment methods the focus will change from a minimum requirement of clinical hours to an attainment of competencies[5] as was discussed earlier in this chapter through AACN's APRN Doctoral-Level Competencies and Progression Indicators.[3] Regardless of the variance in practice hour requirements, your required hours should be well documented as they are required for completion of your program and applying for board certification.

Clinical Documentation

Documentation of clinical hour requirements includes clinical site information as well as preceptors' names, credentials, and practice addresses. Specific documentation related to procedures is also required and should be documented as you progress through your program (Table 1-2). If your future employer is a hospital or medical center, an Ongoing Professional Practice Evaluation (OPPE) report and a Focused Professional Practice Evaluation (FPPE) report will be performed related to your procedural skills requested and for their continued performance.[6] OPPE/FPPE are methods used by hospitals to make decisions regarding privileging. These reports are utilized for initial privileging (OPPE) as well as ongoing (FPPE) privileging. This is based on the requirement of assuring that quality and safety of care delivered to patients requires the monitoring of the performance of all practitioners.[6] This same professional practice evaluation is utilized for physician providers, physician assistants, etc. Per the Joint Commission (2016) OPPE is the screening tool used to evaluate all practitioners who have been granted privileges and to identify those clinicians who might be delivering an unacceptable quality of care. The guidelines for the initial acceptable number of procedures performed as well as the number of procedures required for renewal are frequently defined by national certifying bodies (e.g., American Thoracic Society). FPPE is the follow-up process used to continually evaluate the practitioners' safe performance and quality. The number of required procedures for initial privileging may be more than what is required for renewal. This number may vary from one healthcare institution to another.

Having an initial log with didactic/lab documentation of your requested procedures will be a great starting point (Table 1-2). You can continue to build on this log when you begin practicing as a new NP.

Some academic programs utilize software programs (i.e., Typhon) to record student clinical hours as well as procedures.[7] If you do not utilize such a software program, early on you could develop a spreadsheet on which to continually track your required hours.

Keeping this documentation current during your program is critical and saves time when it is necessary to complete this information at graduation or to supply to a future employer when seeking your first position post graduation (Table 1-3). Keeping the data current on an ongoing basis will also minimize omitting a procedure or skill that you performed during your NP program. You will find that most program faculty require these logs to be updated within 24 of completion of your clinical day.

TABLE 1-2

Sample Procedure Log

Procedure	Location	Lab setting	Clinical setting
Suturing	Pigs feet	May 2019	July 2020
	Scalp laceration		July 2020
	Forearm		
Central line insertion	Right subclavian	October 2019	September 2020
	Left subclavian		October 2020

TABLE 1-3

Sample Clinical Site Log

Date	Practice site	Site address	Preceptor name	Credential	Clinical hours
September– December 2019	Lee Medical Center	104 Main St. Long, VA. 12345	Jane Doe John Smith	RN, ACNP MD	80 60
				Total hours	
				140	

The information regarding your clinical practice site is also required by the certification organizations such as the American Nurses Credentialing Center (ANCC) and the American Academy of Nurse Practitioners Certification Program (AANPCP)[7] in addition to other certification bodies.

Month-by-Month Planner

Most recommendations state that the final preparations and a national board certification examination study plan should start 6 months prior to graduation.[9] The final months before graduation quickly become extremely busy. During this time, you will be completing your program with all of its requirements, preparing for your national board certification examination, interviewing for your new role, and hopefully taking some time to enjoy graduation. You may want to develop a month-by-month planner to assist you in this transition from student NP to graduate NP. You can also utilize your planner to organize the study sessions for your national board certification examination. Often students form study groups to enhance the certification board preparation. You should begin to formulate a tentative date of when you anticipate taking your national board certification examination as well as which national certifying organization you will utilize. Formulating this tentative date will enable you to better project to future employers your anticipated start date in your new role.

NATIONAL BOARD CERTIFICATION EXAMINATION

Determining what national board certifying organization you will choose for your examination should also begin in your final semester of your academic program. You will want to carefully evaluate each certifying body that is specific to your NP specialty.[8] Discuss your options with your program faculty. You will want to become familiar with their specific requirements and application process. Although not on the forefront of your planning, review their certification renewal requirements as well. The certifying organization you choose will depend on your specific NP program. There are specific certifying organizations for Adult-Gerontology Primary Care versus Family or Women's Health Nurse Practitioners. The process of applying for certification can be confusing and you should seek advice from your faculty and the website(s) for specific questions. The NP program director's signature will also be required on your application. If you are not already a member of the national organization that you will be testing with, you may want to consider joining prior to registering for the examination. Student memberships are usually discounted (e.g., American Academy of Nurse Practitioners).

NATIONAL BOARD CERTIFICATION REVIEW COURSE

Several organizations offer board certification review courses. These courses may be in person or through textbooks or CDs.

By now you know your individual learning style and can choose a review method(s) that will work best for you. Practice-test examinations are also offered may be used by NP programs to help students evaluate their learning needs. The questions can also be taken individually on your own time. The practice-test examinations provide an excellent way for the student NP to gauge their preparedness for the national board certification examination as well as providing information regarding areas that more study emphasis is needed.

Two well-known organizations are Barkley & Associates[10] and Fitzgerald Health Education Associates.[11] Barkley & Associates[10] have a variety of "diagnostic readiness tests" available to faculty for their students. The 3P's Assessment test is for first-year NPs—examining pharmacology, physical assessment, and advanced pathophysiology. There is also a 100-item Diagnostic Readiness Test that is population-foci specific for a nominal charge. Fitzgerald's also provides sample exams and test questions. There is also a continuing education (CE) tracker for all of your CE activities. Both organizations provide various examination preparation tests and review books. The review courses are comprehensive and evidence-based. Each site presents their data on successful passage rates. They also list their specific guidelines and costs if a retest is required. Group discounts are also available. This is where you might find it helpful to discuss with your core classmates what exam they are taking. Reviewing each website and consulting with faculty will enable you to choose the program that best fits your needs.

Summary

Planning for graduation starts with the decision to become an NP and continues throughout your NP program. Understanding your specific APRN role is essential. Up-to-date and thorough documentation of clinical hours, courses, and clinical sites is a necessary requirement. It is easier if you begin to keep a database of this information on day one and continually update it than it is to try to reconstruct one at the end of your program. Choosing the latter method leads to missing critical details. Determining what national board certifying body you will choose should be a joint decision between you and the faculty in your specific program. Initiating these steps at the beginning of your program will save you time and energy as you complete your program and plan for graduation.

References

1. APRN Consensus Model. www.ncsbn.org. Accessed June 12, 2018.
2. National Organization of Nurse Practitioner Faculties. http://www.nonpf.org; http://www.npcourses.com/events-live-course-schedule. Accessed June 12, 2018.
3. American Associations of Colleges of Nursing. www.aacnnursing.org/education-Resources/Curriculum-Guidelines. Accessed August 20, 2018.
4. Commission on Collegiate Nursing Education (CCNE). www.aacnnursing./CCNE. Accessed August 21, 2018.
5. AACN—Criteria for Evaluation of Nurse Practitioner Programs 2012. http://www.aacn.nche.edu. Accessed June 12, 2018.
6. The Joint Commission. http://www.jointcomission.org. Accessed June 12, 2018.
7. Typhon Group Healthcare Solutions. http://www.typhongroup.com. Accessed June 12, 2018.
8. Dillon, D. & Hoyson, P. (2013). From Graduation to Employment: A Guide for the New Nurse Practitioner. *The Journal for Nurse Practitioners,* 9 (1) 55–59.
9. American Nurses Credentialing Center. http://www.nursecredentialing.org. Accessed June 12, 2018.
10. Barkley & Associates. https://npcourses.com. Accessed July 2, 2018.
11. Fitzgerald Health Education Associates. *The Journal for Nurse Practitioners*, 312–315. https://fhea.com. Accessed June 12, 2018.

2

National Board
Certification Exam

Forty-seven states require nurse practitioners to have a master's degree which then enables them to sit for a national board certification examination. Most states require an active registered nurse (RN) license in addition to a national board certification to enable to practice as an NP. The RN and NP license must be issued from the same state. If you are planning on practicing in another state after graduation, you will want to apply for an RN license in that state as well. In 2015 the National Council of the State Boards of Nursing approved the APRN Compact which allows an advanced practice RN to hold one multistate license with a privilege to practice in other compact states. In 2015 the APRN Compact became available for specific states (Idaho, Wyoming, and North Dakota).[1] This is a continuing process with more states anticipating participation in a multi-state licensure process.

Currently there are seven National Certifying Organizations (Table 2-1).

As mentioned previously, have a discussion with your faculty regarding which certification organization is appropriate for your specific educational tract. The APRN Consensus Model requires alignment in licensure, education, and certification. Always review the specific certification organization websites for the most up-to-date information. Review the specific application packet completely. The application may be completed on paper or online. Some of the certifying bodies have completely eliminated a paper submission. Before submission, review your application for accuracy and completeness. Utilize checklists if they are provided. It is helpful to have all of your documentation organized prior to completing the necessary paperwork.

COURSE COMPLETION INFORMATION

You will need specific information on courses completed, course number, credit hours, and year taken (this is where those documentation logs you completed come in handy). You may have

TABLE 2-1

National Certifying Organizations

Certifying organization	Website	Certification examinations offered
American Academy of Nurse Practitioners Certification Board (AANPCB)	ww.aanpcert.org	Board, Family Nurse Practitioner Adult-Gerontology Primary Care Emergency Nurse Practitioner
American Association of Critical Care Nurses (AACN)	www.aacn.org	Acute Care (recertification only), Adult-Gerontology Acute Care Nurse Practitioner
American Midwifery Certification Board	www.amcbmidwife.org	Certified Midwife Certified Nurse Midwife
American Nurses Credentialing Center (ANCC)	www.nursecredentialing.org	Acute Care (recertification only), Adult (recertification only), Adult-Gerontology Acute Care, Adult-Gerontology Primary Care, Adult Psych-Mental Health, Psychiatric -Mental Health (across the lifespan) Emergency, Family, Gerontology, Pediatric Primary Care, and School Nurse Practitioners

(Continued)

TABLE 2-1

National Certifying Organizations *(Continued)*

Certifying organization	Website	Certification examinations offered
National Certification Corporation (NCC)	www.nccwebsite.org/ certification-exams.org	Women's Health Care and Neonatal Nurse Practitioners
Oncology Nursing Certification Corporation	www.oncc.org	Advanced Oncology Certified Nurse Practitioner
Pediatric Nursing Certification Board (PNCB)	www.pncb.org	Acute and Primary Care Pediatric Nurse Practitioner

this information in your portfolio as well. Each NP specialty has a specific minimum number of clinical hours required for their national board certification (e.g., Adult-Gerontology 500 clinical hours). University programs may require additional hours to complete their specific program. This clinical hour requirement can vary from university to university in the same program specialty. For example, your program might require 700 clinical hours to complete the program and graduate, even though the certification body states a minimum of 500 clinical hours is required. A different university might require 650 hours for the same program specialty. You can always be over the amount of clinical hours. Usually a photocopy of your current RN license or a copy of the Board of Nursing verification website listing is also required. Specific details on your clinical hours including precepting practice site, address, site specialty, preceptor's name and credentials are required as well as the total clock hours spent at each site.

OFFICIAL GRADE TRANSCRIPTS

Official grade transcripts will need to be requested by you from your university's registrar office. Some universities require an associated fee for these transcripts. Often your request is free. The official transcripts will be submitted from/by the university registrar's office in a separate sealed envelope to a specified address when they are available. Official transcripts will have the university insignia, degree completed, and degree conferred on them as well. You may want to check with your university's registrar's office on how soon after final grade posting the transcripts are available. There may also be a Validation of Education Form that needs to be signed by your faculty (e.g., ANCC). A copy of the completed application should be kept for your records. Completing the application early allows time if corrections or completion of the application is needed.

NAME CHANGING

If you are anticipating a name change by the time you take your certification exam, there are some additional things to consider. On the day you present to the testing center for your exam you will need two forms of identification that match the name on the application **exactly**. Allow yourself enough time to have your driver's license or other picture form of identification changed prior to your testing date.

APPLICATION FEE

All applications require an application fee that is submitted at the time of your application. Often there are significant discounts available if you are a member of the certifying organization. Student member rates are usually lower. So the time to join these professional organizations is while you are still a student.

The two most widely used certifying organizations are the American Nurses Credentialing Center (ANCC)[2] and the American Academy of Nurse Practitioners (AANP).[3] The American Association of Critical Care Nurses (AACN) also has a certification examination available for the adult-gerontology acute care nurse practitioner.[4] There are cost differences between these organizations and their initial certification examination as well differences in the application process.

EXAM PREPARATION

It is recommended that studying for your national board certification should start 6 months prior to graduation.[2] There are various review courses available as well as textbooks and CDs to assist with the preparation process. The more common review courses are offered by Barkley & Associates[5] and Fitzgerald Health Education Associates.[6] The Advanced Practice Education Associates (APEA)[7] also offers review courses for the FNP and Adult-Gerontology Primary Care NP. At this point in time, you know what method of study works best for you. Some students prefer the study group method. Others prefer individual study time. Most of the certifying organizations also provide sample questions or self-assessment exams to help guide the studying process. They may also have available for you study materials/books. You should take advantage of the resources that are available through the various certifying agencies (i.e., practice questions and other study materials).

AMERICAN ACADEMY OF NURSE PRACTITIONERS CERTIFICATION PROGRAM (AANPCB)

The AANPCB has been an online process since 2010. In 2017, the American Academy of Nurse Practitioners Certification Program (AANPCP) changed their name to the American Academy of Nurse Practitioners Certification Board (AANPCB). They offer certification examinations for Adult Nurse Practitioners (ANP-C) (retired in December 2016), Adult-Gerontology Primary Care Nurse Practitioners (AGNP-C), and Family Nurse Practitioners (FNP-C) and Emergency NP (ENP-C). Paper applications are available for those candidates who are unable to utilize the web-based application process. A nonrefundable paper application processing fee is automatically charged for all paper applications, regardless of the delivery method (e.g., email, mail, and fax). There is no charge for receipt of documents or RN license faxed, emailed, or mailed.[3] Applicants may sit for the examination after completion of didactic courses and clinical practice hours.

Applicants may go online and completed a certification profile. AANPCB provides notification to the candidate once all documentation has been approved. AANPCB also notifies PSI services of the candidate's eligibility to test. Within 24 hours of notification, PSI will send the candidate an eligibility confirmation email which will provide you with your **Eligibility ID Number**, grant the 120-day testing window, and provide important instructions for scheduling your appointment at a PSI testing center.[8] Your application status can be reviewed online at anytime. Once you have received your eligibility to test notification from both AANPCB and PSI, the fastest and most convenient way to schedule your exam is online by accessing the PSI scheduling website at https://psiexams.com. Candidates may also contact a PSI customer service representative at 800-892-5473 during PSI hours of operation. These testing centers are located throughout the United States. If the testing is not completed within this time frame, candidates will be required to resubmit their application as well as appropriate fees.[8]

In 2013, AANPPCB partnered with a third party service to provide a computer-based testing practice examination to examination candidates. The practice exams are for the Family Nurse Practitioner, Adult Nurse Practitioner (was retired in December 2016), the Adult-Gerontology Primary Care Practice, and the Emergency NP. There are 3 versions of the FNP practice test, two versions of the Adult-Gerontology NP, and one version of the Emergency NP practice test.[3] There is also no verification fee for the notification of certification to be sent by AANPCB to the State Board of Nursing.

At the completion of your exam you will be notified of a preliminary instructor–passed/not passed printout. Official score letters are mailed within 2-3 weeks if the candidate's application is complete and a final transcript showing degree awarded has been received and processed by AANPCB.[3]

AMERICAN NURSES CREDENTIALING CENTER

ANCC offers certification examinations for the following nurse practitioners: Acute Care NP (ACNP-BC-retired-re-certification renewal only), Adult Nurse NP (ANP-BC-retired-recertification-renewal only), Adult-Gerontology Acute Care NP (AGACNP-BC), Gerontology Primary Care NP (AGPCNP-BC), Psychiatric-Mental Health NP (APMHNP-BC), Family NP (FNP-BC), Gerontological NP (GNP-BC), Pediatric Primary Care NP (PPCNP-BC), Psychiatric Mental Health NP (Across the Lifespan) (PMHNP-BC), and School NP (SNP-BC). They also offer the following two specialty NP certifications in Diabetes Management and Emergency NP. Test content outlines are available on the ANCC website. ANCC has a certification-general testing and renewal handbook also available on their website.

ANCC's website states that the candidate will usually receive notification that your application was received within 2 weeks. Within 6 weeks from the time you mailed your application, you will receive your eligibility notice or Authorization to Test (ATT) or a letter requesting additional information. The eligibility notice gives the candidate a 90-day window in which to schedule and take the certification examination. You are recommended to schedule as soon as possible to ensure you get your desired date and time. If for some reason you are unable to test during the 90-day window, you may, one time only, request a new 90-day testing window. This new testing window must begin less than 6 months from the last day of the initial testing window. If you do not test during your new testing window, you will need to reapply as a new applicant, meet any new eligibility requirements, and pay all applicable fees. To make this request, you must complete the Testing Window Re-Assignment Request form at www.nursecredentialing.org/ReAssignmentRequestForm.aspx.2

ANCC certification candidates may be authorized to sit for the examination after all coursework is completed and prior to degree conferral. ANCC will retain the candidate's exam result and will issue certification on the date the requested documents are received, all eligibility requirements are met, and a passing result is on file.[2]

Prometric test centers[9] (www.prometric.com/ANCC) are utilized for all ANCC certification exam testing. When you have all of your appropriate documentation and are ready to take the exam, use the Prometric test center directory to find the closest location. Their website has specific information related to the testing day (www.prometric.com/ANCC). The test drive allows candidates to walk through, on a practical basis, all check-in and testing procedures that occur at the test center on test day. The charge of $30.00 is incurred for the test drive option. Enrollment is through the same website.

After you have taken your examination, you will receive a copy of your results instantly at the testing site. If you successfully complete the examination, you will receive a certificate and pin within 4 weeks. ANCC does not automatically send verification to you, the State Board of Nursing, or to your employer.[2] This means that you must request an official copy to be sent to your specific State Board of Nursing and to your employer. There may be a corresponding fee associated.

AMERICAN ASSOCIATION OF CRITICAL CARE NURSES

In 2007 AACN began offering the Acute Care Nurse Practitioner Certification (ACNPC-AG).[4] In 2013, AACN Certification Corporation launched a Consensus Model-based adult-gerontology

ACNP certification examination.[4] Practice questions are available on the website. A practice ACNPC-AG exam questions text is available free when you apply for the ACNPC-AG certification examination. Further specifics on testing are available on the AACN website.[4] You may also access the AACN exam handbook on this website. The certification examination is computer-based and is offered at 300 PSI testing. testing sites across the United States.[10] AMP is a nationally known testing center. Candidates are allowed 3½ hours to complete the examination. At the completion of the exam the proctor will provide you with your official exam score.[11]

NATIONAL CERTIFICATION CORPORATION (NCC)

NCC is the organization utilized by Neonatal Nurse Practitioners (NNP-BC) and Women's Health Care Nurse Practitioners (WHNP-BC) for their specialty certification.[12] The certification examination is computer-based and is offered at AMP/PSI testing sites across the United States.[10] Candidates schedule their own exam testing. An examination handbook is available on line on their website (www.nccwebsite.org/cert-exams).

An application for certification may be submitted at any time. The review and approval process can take up to 4 weeks. Prior to taking the examination, you will be allowed to take a practice exam. No results are provided immediately after testing for any format. Official results are mailed from NCC within 15 days days of the exam administration date. The candidate is not certified until the exam results are received in the mail. This is a 3 hour examination with 175 questions.

PEDIATRIC NURSING CERTIFICATION BOARD (PNCB)

PNCB is the certifying organization for Primary Care Pediatric Nurse Practitioners (CNP-PC) and Acute Care Pediatric Nurse

Practitioners (CNP-AC).[13] PNCB delivers its examination through prometric testing centers (http://prometric.com/PNCB). They provide the following resources to candidates which include a practice exam test, test-taking strategies module, and examination resources specific to the specialty certification. The examination is web-based and must be taken within a 90-day time frame. This date is provided on the postcard and eligibility letter that the candidate receives. Testing is completed at a Prometric testing center[9] and is scheduled by the candidate. The 90-day testing window may be extended, on a one-time basis, if specific criteria are met. An additional registration fee is required for the extension. The CPCP and CPN are timed exams with 175 multiple-choice questions. Twenty-five of the questions are non-scored test items and are randomly distributed throughout the exam. At completion of your exam you report to the proctor to receive your personal, preliminary exam results of exam status = pass or exam status = fail. Official examination results will be mailed within 10 days from PNCB. An official certificate with certification number, a wall certificate, and additional material are mailed within 4-6 weeks following your testing date. Specific details regarding the certification process are available on the PNCB website.[13]

THE NEED TO CANCEL AND RESCHEDULE

Life events and illness can and do happen and there may be a need to cancel and reschedule your certification examination. The testing centers require a 2-day notification of a cancellation prior to your scheduled test date. You must call the specific number listed on the website to cancel and reschedule your appointment. You will also be required to reschedule your testing if you appear at the test site after the examination has started or if you do not present proper identification when you arrive at the testing center. It is best to refer to the specific testing site for details if the need to cancel and reschedule should arise.

SPECIAL ACCOMMODATIONS

As per the website of PSI (https://candidate.psiexams.com) all centers are equipped to provide access in accordance with the American with Disabilities Act (ADA) of 1990, and exam accommodations will be made in meeting a candidate's needs. A Special Accommodation Request Application Form needs to be completed prior to scheduling your examination. The form is available at http://www.aanpcert.org. The website stresses not scheduling your examination until your documentation has been received and processed by the PSI special accommodations department. The application will be reviewed and the candidate will be contacted by a PSI special accommodations team member within 48 to 72 hours to arrange necessary accommodations.

TEST CENTER SECURITY

Testing centers vary in their security requirements. Do not bring any unnecessary material with you. The following items may be inspected during the check-in process—eyeglasses, jewelry, and other accessories to look for cameras that could be used to capture test content.[9] These checks are performed at check-in and upon return from breaks. Jewelry outside of wedding and engagement rings is prohibited. Hair accessories and ties are subject to inspection. If items are deemed inappropriate you will be asked to remove them and store them in your locker. Some states require Electronic Biometric capture (fingerprinting) prior to or on the day of testing. Metal detector scanning may also be required. Please read instructions clearly.

TESTING DAY

Testing sites request you to arrive at least 15-30 minutes before your scheduled testing time. It is ideal if you can do a "trial run" to the testing site to determine its exact location as well as the approximate time it will take you to arrive. If you are not able to do this in advance of your testing date, allow additional time on your exact date to allow for traffic pattern changes, detours, as well as a possible "wrong turn." Remember to allow time for parking and walking to the centers. Candidates who arrive late for their scheduled testing (or miss their scheduled examination appointment), or arrive without the required documentation, will not be able to take their examination as scheduled and will need to reschedule. This policy is standard for all the testing sites.

Specific requirements for each testing center are available on their websites. You must bring two forms of required documentation that will match the name on your certification exam application. One form of identification usually requires a photo. The eligibility notice or ATT letter must also be brought with you that day. Do not bring unnecessary items with you. (ie. phone, calculator, food or drink). It is actually better if you don't bring anything with you. Any belongings you bring into the testing center will be secured in a locker until exam completion.

You will be given an introductory tutorial before you take the actual examination. This will allow you to practice using the keys, answering questions, and reviewing your answers. The examination questions will appear on the screen one at a time. You will have an opportunity to return to your questions for review, provided the test time has not ran out. The length of the examination and total number of questions may vary depending on the certifying agency. The ANCC certification exam for Family Nurse Practitioner, for example, allows 3.5 hours to answer 175 questions. This includes 25 practice questions which are not scored.[2] AACN, ANCC, and the PNCB certification examinations each have 175 multiple-choice questions.[11-13] One hundred and fifty of the questions are scored and 25 are used to gather statistical data on item performance for future examinations.

SUCCESSFUL COMPLETION OF CERTIFICATION EXAMINATION

After successful completion of your certification examination, you will receive a preliminary result at the time of testing. The official results will arrive in the mail several weeks after your testing. With successful completion of the certification examination you will have new initials after your name. These initials will vary depending on the certifying examination which you took as well as the specific certifying agency.

WHAT TO DO WITH ALL THE INITIALS

ANCC[2] has recommendations for placement of the certifications and provides a great handout with the specific details. The sequence is usually based on the order of which credential is least likely to be taken away in descending order. The first credential listed after your legal name should be your highest level of education (e.g., PhD, DNP, or MSN). A degree is usually permanent and in most instances cannot be taken away. It is not considered necessary to list your master's degree if you have attained a doctoral degree unless both degrees are in different areas (i.e., PhD, MBA). This is because a PhD "trumps" them all.[14] The second credential is your RN license. Licensure is followed by specific state designations. The Consensus Model is encouraging states to adopt the title of APRN, but check with your specific state board of nursing on advanced practice nursing titles. The third credential is your national certification (e.g., AGACNP-BC, FNP-BC). These can be taken away if not renewed. The fourth credential could be a certification that denotes a degree of expertise in that specific area (e.g., CCRN, CHFN). These credentials are typically placed in the order in which they were earned. The most recent credential being last. Initials denoting a nursing fellowship should be the last initials displayed in your formal title. Most practitioners utilize this complete set of initials on letterhead, business cards, and other such professional documents. While you want to be recognized for the achievements you have, you want to avoid your title looking like alphabet soup.

It is important to remember that the only credential you are required to use is the one required by your specific state board of nursing. This credential must also be on prescriptions, documentation, and medical records. As always, familiarize yourself with your specific board of nursing requirements.

UNSUCCESSFUL COMPLETION OF CERTIFICATION EXAMINATION

Of course, a successful pass rate is desirable at the time of the first test. Unfortunately, this does not always happen. You will receive a copy of test results prior to leaving the exam testing center. Each certifying organization has specific recommendations and requirements on retesting. They will specify the timing and educational requirements (if noted) that must be met prior to rescheduling your examination. In most instances there is a time frame you must meet before rescheduling your retake exam. This will allow you time to focus on designated areas and in some instances complete required continuing education before retesting. Board certification exam scores and passage rates are available at each school of nursing as well as an average pass rate for each of the certifying organizations. Some students utilized the certifying organizations passage rate as a barometer for which exam to sit for.

Summary

The culmination of your academic success is measured by your completion of your national board certification examination. Understanding the process, paying attention to details, and preparing yourself are ways to make this a less stressful and a successful experience. Taking the time to review the process as well as study preparation will be time well spent.

References

1. National Council State Boards of Nursing APRN Compact (May 2015). https://www.ncsbn.org/aprn-compact.htm. Accessed September 2, 2020.
2. American Nurse Credentialing Center (ANCC). http://www.nursecredentialing.org. Accessed September 2, 2020.
3. American Academy of Nurse Practitioners Certification Program. http://www.aanpcert.org/ptistore/control/index. Accessed September 2, 2020.
4. American Association of Critical Care Nurses Certification Corporation. http://www.aacn.org. Accessed September 2, 2020.
5. Barkley & Associates. https://npcourses.com. Accessed September 2, 2020.
6. Fitzgerald Health Education Associates. https://fhea.com. Accessed September 2, 2020.
7. Advanced Practice Education Association. APEA. www.apea.com.
8. PSI Testing Centers. www.psiexams.com/ANCC. Accessed September 2, 2020.
9. Prometric Testing Center. http://www.prometric.com. Accessed June 12, 2018.
10. AMP. http://www.goAMP.com. Accessed September 2, 2020.
11. Nurses, A. A. (2016). *AACN Certification Exam Policy Handbook* (p. 19). Aliso Viejo: AACN. Accessed September 2, 2020.
12. National Certification Corporation. http://www.nccwebsite.org/Certification/Certification-Exams.aspx. Accessed September 2, 2020.
13. Pediatric Nursing Certification Board. http://www.pncb.org/ptistore/control/index. Accessed Accessed September 2, 2020.
14. Menski, J. (2018). What's the Right Way to List Your Nursing Credentials? *Nurs.com*. 10.

3

Applying for State Licensure

INTRODUCTION

Licensure is required by many professions as a means of protecting the public from harm. It is licensure that sets the minimal qualifications and competencies for safe, entry-level practitioners. The general public may not have sufficient information and experience to identify an unqualified healthcare provider, and is therefore vulnerable to unsafe and incompetent practitioners. A license issued by a government entity (e.g., the state Board of Nursing [BON]) provides this assurance to the public that the nurse has met these predetermined standards.[1]

Successful completion of your board certification exam enables you to submit your application to your specific state BON for your license as an NP. Certification is granted by the national board certification organizations after successful completion of your certification examination. Nurse practitioner licensure is granted by individual states. So just to be sure you have this clear—your board certification is not your NP license. The NP license is granted by your state. Professional certification and licensure are required by NPs in almost every state. There is significant variability between states' laws on specific criteria for licensure. Nurse practitioner requirements are set at the state level.

Individual states may approve certifying agencies or approve individual certification examinations. Other states may defer to organizations that accredit certification agencies. They may reference the National Commission for Certifying Agencies and/or the American Board of Nursing Specialties.[2]

Some state boards allow the NP graduate to practice for a limited time after graduation, by issuing a temporary permit, pending certification. Defined timelines are identified and strictly enforced. Certification examination failure invalidates a temporary credential.

Referring to the state BON website in your specific state is recommended. Nursing Licensure.org is an excellent website to get specific information regarding your RN and NP license.[2] On this site you will find detailed instructions for completion and list of required materials to submit.

REQUIREMENTS

Individual states regulate licensure requirements. All 50 states require NPs to have a registered nurse (RN) license. Forty states require NPs to have master's degrees. Forty-five states require NPs to have obtained national certification.[3]

APPLYING FOR LICENSURE

Unlike your RN licensure, there is no NCLEX-RN exam for the nurse practitioner to achieve licensure at the state level. The NP certification examination is used by most states to determine the competency of a candidate. After successful completion of your certification examination you must then apply to your state BON to be licensed. One certifying organization, the American Nurses Credentialing Center (ANCC) will notify the state BON at no charge if you have completed the state (BON) notification form. All of the certifying organizations provide a means for your examination results to be sent to your specific BON. These details are outlined on their individual websites.

THE APRN CONSENSUS MODEL

In alignment with the APRN Consensus Model your license to practice as an NP should match with your educational preparation. Some states have made legislative changes to conform to the National Council of State Board of Nursing APRN Consensus model. As of 2020, 36 states and US territory Boards of Nursing have enacted the Consensus Model.[4] The adoption of the Consensus Model for Advanced Practice Nursing[5] has enabled plans to go into action to make requirements more consistent and licenses more portable, to train Advanced Practice Registered Nurses (APRNs) well, and then allow them to practice to the full extent of their education and training.[2] The APRN Consensus Model defines advanced practice registered nurse practice, describes the APRN regulatory model, identifies the titles to be used, defines specialty, describes the emergence of new roles and population foci, and presents strategies for implementation.[6] In the APRN Consensus Model, licensure is defined as granting the authority to practice. One of the foundational requirements for licensure is to license APRNs as independent practitioners with no regulatory requirements for collaboration, direction, or supervision.[6]

Despite the Consensus Model recommendations there are still challenges ahead of us. Some of the challenges are that not all APRNs are regulated by Boards of Nursing, states still use different terminology for the APRN roles (i.e., CNP vs. APRN), have different legislation for each of the four APRN roles, do not all require graduate education, and do not have full practice authority (FPA) for any APRNs.

Full Practice Authority

Nurse practitioner licensure continues to change. In this instance, change is a good thing. FPA, as defined by the American Association of Nurse Practitioners (AANP), is "the collection of state practice and licensure laws that allow for nurse practitioners to evaluate patients, diagnose, order and interpret diagnostic tests, initiate and manage treatments—including prescribing medications—under the exclusive licensure authority of the State Board of Nursing."[7] FPA is the model recommended by the Institute of Medicine and National Council of State Boards of Nursing. Currently 23 states, the District of Columbia, and Guam and the Marianas Islands have FPA and more states have legislation currently pending, for example, Pennsylvania.[8] This legislation is changing the licensure application process in many states.

Nurse practitioners are encouraged to be active in their respective state organizations to work together for legislation that supports FPA in their state (Fig. 3-1).[7]

FIGURE 3-1 AANP 2021 Nurse Practitioner State Practice Environment

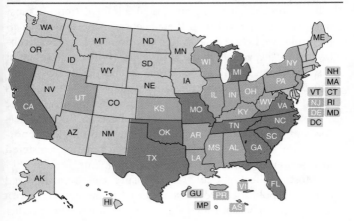

Full Practice: State practice and licensure laws permit all NPs to evaluate patients; diagnose, order and interpret diagnostic tests; and initiate and manage treatments, including prescribing medications and controlled substances, under the exclusive licensure authority of the state board of nursing. This is the model recommended by the National Academy of Medicine, formerly called the Institute of Medicine, and the National Council of State Boards of Nursing.

Reduced Practice: State practice and licensure laws reduce the ability of NPs to engage in at least one element of NP practice. State law requires a career-long regulated collaborative agreement with another health provider in order for the NP to provide patient care, or it limits the setting of one or more elements of NP practice.

Restricted Practice: State practice and licensure laws restrict the ability of NPs to engage in at least one element of NP practice. State law requires career-long supervision, delegation or team management by another health provider in order for the NP to provide patient care.

(Reprinted with permission from the American Association of Nurse Practitioners.)
Updated 1.2021

STATE LICENSING

An active RN license is a prerequisite for obtaining an NP license in most states. The state BON of each individual state is the best source for licensing and practice information.[2] In most instances, the NPs will hold their license in the same state in which they are licensed as an RN. RN licensure and NP licensure are not always held in the same state. Approximately half of US states belong to the nurse license compact at the RN level.[2] In 2015 the APRN Compact became available for specific states (Idaho, Wyoming, and North Dakota). The purpose of the APRN Compact is to decrease redundancies in the consideration and issuance of APRN licensure; and to provide opportunities for interstate practice by advanced practice registered nurses who meet uniform licensure requirements.[9]

Most applications for NP licensure can be completed online. An application fee is also required. Some states require a recent photo to be submitted with the application. The specifics on size, color, age of photo are delineated on the website. Most states require proof of certification as a nurse practitioner to be forwarded directly from the certifying organization. A copy of official grade transcripts directly from your academic institution is often required as well. Again, specific details should be obtained from the state BON website for the specific state in which you are seeking licensure as an NP. The state BON website enables you to check the status of your application as well. Some sites list items that have been received or are still pending to enable you to follow up as necessary.

PRESCRIPTIVE AUTHORITY

As a part of their daily practice more than 95% of nurse practitioners prescribe medications and those working in a full-time practice write an average of 23 prescriptions per day. NPs have prescriptive authority in all 50 states including Washington, DC.[10]

In order to prescribe, certain states require an additional application must also be submitted for prescribing or prescriptive authority. The specific details related to the application will be available on the state BON website as well. Requirements for prescribing usually include a graduate-level pharmacology course. Most advanced pharmacology courses for nurse practitioners are approximately 4 to 5 credit hours. There is often a time requirement placed on the course as well, for example, must be taken within 2 to 5 years prior to the application for prescriptive authority. If for some reason you find yourself outside of this window, there are online continuing education courses in pharmacology that could be used to meet this requirement. These courses are usually 45 contact hours in duration. Prior to enrolling in the course you will want to check with your state BON to be certain the course meets their requirements. This option is less expensive and more convenient than repeating a university-based pharmacology course. In some states, such as New York, you will also want to submit an application for a Furnishing Number in order to prescribe medications and a DEA application to prescribe controlled substances.11. California issues a furnishing number.

An application fee is also required for the prescriptive authority. There is a separate number associated with this prescribing license. This number must be displayed on all prescriptions. In some instances, this license cannot be applied for until you have established with a collaborating physician and have a practice address. Initial certification may also require an externship period with a certain number of supervised prescribing hours prior to independent prescribing. This requirement of supervised hours varies from state to state. Full prescriptive authority may require 2000 or more mentored/supervised hours. Some states allow another NP with prescriptive authority to monitor you and sign off on hours during this period. They may be allowed to mentor the entire process or be restricted to a predetermined hour requirement. Your collaborating physician is responsible for mentoring hours as well. If the state does not have a specific form for documenting these hours you may want to create your own log. The documentation log should be specific as to the name of the provider who performed the monitoring as well as the total hours with each provider. Each practitioner should become extremely familiar with their specific state's legislation on prescribing. There are also pharmacology continuing education hours that are assigned to prescriptive authority renewal. These are in addition to the continuing education hours required for RN and NP license renewals. Once your NP license number and prescribing number are approved they will be listed on the state BON's verification website with the associated expiration date.

CONTROLLED SUBSTANCES

Twenty-eight states and the District of Columbia allow full practice authority.[7] In these states NPs have similar prescriptive authority as a physician. In the 16 states with reduced practice authority, NPs are required to have a collaborative agreement with a physician(s) to gain prescriptive privileges. Often a requirement for prescribing both controlled and non-controlled drugs, the collaborating physician must be in the same specialty as the NP. Some states require consultation and referral plans to prescribe Schedule II to III controlled drugs. These privileges usually have limitations on the medications that the NP is allowed to prescribe. As of today, five states do not allow the prescribing of Schedule II medications by NPs. These states include Georgia, Oklahoma, and West Virginia. Arkansas and Missouri limit NPs to prescribing hydrocodone combination products only.[10] In July 2018, South Carolina NPs received authority to prescribe a 2- to 5-day supply of Schedule II medications.[12]

In order to prescribe controlled substances, you must apply for a DEA (Drug Enforcement Agency) number.[12] The DEA is part of the US Department of Justice and is responsible for regulating licensing for controlled substances. You may apply for your DEA license online (http://www.deadiversion.usdoj.gov) once you have received your NP license and have a practice address. The DEA number must be displayed on all prescriptions written by an NP.

NPs should remember that in specific states a DEA license is also accompanied by an additional prescriptive authority number application. Providers should be very familiar with their state's requirements. States, such as Pennsylvania, require a separate state-level application for prescribing controlled substances.[8] This is sometimes referred to as a state CDS (Controlled Dangerous Substance) number. The DEA is a federally issued license and does not supersede a state's specific prescribing requirements. The DEA is necessary for prescribing controlled substances and must be renewed every 3 years. DEA Form 224a is the application form for mid-level providers. The 3-year renewable fee is $731.00. Some employers may include the cost of a DEA license in you benefit package.

There are six sections of the online registration process. You will need to have your social security number, business address, phone number, and email address. You must also furnish a valid and active state license(s). Due to the national opioid crisis, most states now require specific pharmacology education and continuing education requirements in order to prescribe controlled substances.

PRESCRIPTION DRUG MONITORING PROGRAMS

Forty-nine states, the District of Columbia, and St. Louis County, MO, require that providers (NPs, PAs, and physicians) participate in a prescription drug monitoring program (PDMP) when prescribing Schedule II medications.[13] The DEA is not involved with the administration of any state PDMP. The PDMP is a statewide electronic database that collects designated data on substances dispensed in the state. Each individual state designates the state agency that will oversee its PDMP. They may be monitored by the pharmacy board, department of health, or state law enforcement. A current list of states contacts is maintained at www.nascsa.org/rxMonitoring.htm.

The purposes of a PDMP are as follows:

- Support access to legitimate medical use of controlled substances
- Identify and deter or prevent drug abuse and diversion
- Facilitate and encourage the identification, intervention with, and treatment of persons addicted to prescription drugs
- Inform public health initiatives through outlining of use and abuse trends, and
- Educate individuals about PDMPs and the use, abuse, and diversion of an addition to prescription drugs[13]

Prescribers are required to access the PDMP any time they are prescribing a controlled substance. With the current status of opioid abuse, misuse, and diversion, the use of PDMPs is felt to be a means of identifying individuals who may be fraudulently obtaining controlled substances from multiple healthcare providers. The PDMP may require a consultation and referral plan to be in place when prescribing Schedule II controlled substances. The PDMP can also be utilized to identify or investigate providers with patterns of inappropriate prescribing and dispensing.

DATA MANAGEMENT

Issuance of an NP certification, state RN and NP license, and a DEA number all come with mandatory renewal periods. Tracking of these new numbers and renewal dates is important so that you do not let any lapse occur in your ability to practice. Developing your own system for this is critical. Do not rely on the certifying organization, state BON, or the DEA to notify you when your renewal is approaching. Not only should you monitor the renewal dates, but be sure you are completing your renewal requirements (i.e., continuing education) along the way. Becoming initially certified and licensed, as well as renewal, is also expensive. Good data management enables you to budget for these practice expenses as well.

Summary

The time from graduation to receiving licensure as an NP depends on several factors. Time must be allowed for the official grade transcripts to be processed. You can inquire through your university's registrar's office as to what is the standard time frame for this process. This is a variable that is dependent upon the university's registrar's office. Some students take "some time off" after graduation knowing that once they are employed their next vacation time may be a year away. Other students may choose to schedule a review course which may be available at a variety of different time intervals. The candidate then may choose to spend time reviewing and culminating that information. It is possible for this time interval to be up to 3 months or longer post graduation. The time from completion of the certification examination to the official posting on the SBON verification website can also vary and may be up to 6 weeks post completion of the examination.

May and June are particularly high-volume months for Boards of Nursing due to the large number of RNs and NPs seeking licensure. These time frames are important for the NP graduate to keep in mind when determining an agreed upon hire date for employment. Some employers may hire an NP who has the issuance of a temporary permit, or is pending the state BON website verification posting, and allow them to initiate the credentialing process. Other employers will not initiate the credentialing process until verification is present on the BON website.

During this time most NP graduates must be in an environment functioning in the role of an RN. There are a few states (e.g., Illinois) that will issue a temporary permit to practice as an advanced practice nurse. The temporary permit in Illinois is issued for a period of 6 months. The graduate must have applied to take a certifying examination. On the application there must be documentation from an approved certifying body indicating the date on which you are scheduled to sit for your examination.[14]

The factors involved in taking your certification examination and applying for state licensure impact when you will determine your availability date for hire by your future employer. Deciding on when you take your certification exam will determine your ability to seek licensure. In most states, this will determine your availability for hiring date.

Data management of these new certification and license numbers is essential so that you are able to practice uninterrupted as well as allot monies in your budget at renewal time. This data management should also include the ongoing monitoring of continuing education requirements and clinical requirements that are also needed for renewal.

References

1. National Council of State Boards of Nursing. https://ncsbn.org/nursing_Licensure.pdf. Accessed September 2, 2020.
2. IOM (2011), The Future of Nursing: Leading Change and Advocacy. Washington, DC:National Academies Press. Accessed September 2, 2020.
3. Buppert, C. (2018). *State Regulation of Nurse Practitioners in Nurse Practitioners Business and Legal Guide* (p. 134). Burlington, MA: Jones & Bartlett.
4. APRN Consensus Work Group & the National Council of State Boards of Registered Nursing APRN Advisory Council. (2008, July 7). Consensus Model for APRN Regulation: Licensure, Accreditation, Certification & Education.

https://www.ncsbn.org/7_23_08 Consensus APRN Final.pdf. Accessed September 2, 2020.

5. National Council of State Boards of Nursing Consensus Model. http://www.ncsbn.org/738htm. Accessed September 2, 2020.

6. American Association of Nurse Practitioners. http://www.aanp.org. Accessed August 27, 2018. September 2, 2020.

7. American Association of Nurse Practitioners. http://www.aanp.org/.../state-practice-environment. Accessed September 2, 2020.

8. Pennsylvania Board of Nursing. http://www.dos.state.pa.us/bpoa/site/default.asp. Accessed.

9. The National Council of State Boards of Nursing. https://www.ncsbn.org/aprn-compact.htm. Accessed September 2, 2020.

10. Herman, J. (2017 June). *Contemporary Clinic.* http://contemporaryclinic.pharmacytimes.com/journals/issue/2017/june2017/prescriptive-authority-update-2017. Accessed September 19, 2017.

11. Department of Consumer Affairs. Nurse Practitioner Furnishing Number Application. Https://www.RN.CA.gov. Accessed September 2, 2020.

12. U.S. Department of Justice Drug Enforcement Administration. http://www.deadiversion.usdoj.gov. Accessed September 2, 2020.

13. The National Alliance for Model State Drug Laws (NAMSDL). http://www.namsl.org. Accessed Accessed September 2, 2020.

14. Illinois Department of Financial and Professional Regulation. https://www.nursinglicensure.org/np-state/illinois-nurse-practitioner.html. Accessed September 2, 2020.

4

The Portfolio

DEVELOPING A PORTFOLIO

A portfolio provides more detail and supplements—not replaces—your resume. Portfolios vary widely, but a key feature is the inclusion of artifacts. Artifacts are tangible objects that demonstrate your work. Examples of artifacts include samples of your work such as history and physicals and progress notes. Faculty often critiques such documents and you should use these examples after you have made the necessary revisions. You will want to be sure that all of this documentation has had patient identifiers removed. Course outlines and syllabi, procedure checklists, etc. that you created by yourself or as part of a team effort, are also important to include. You may also wish to include statements from patients or providers expressing their satisfaction with care you have provided. You may also want to include your diplomas, proof of certifications (i.e., CPR, ACLS, etc.), and licensure in your portfolio. These items should never be the originals but copies only. Portfolios can be paper or electronic; electronic formats include web pages, PDF documents, and even PowerPoint presentations.[1] You may provide a web link to your documents if you have utilized a program such as Typhon[2] to collect your data.

RESUMES AND CURRICULUM VITAE

Both resumes and curriculum vitae (CV) are used when applying for an NP position. There are, however, differences between them. A resume (Table 4-1) is typically shorter and often a one-page synopsis. A CV is more detailed and may be two to three pages in length (Table 4-2). They are not always interchangeable so attention to detail of the instructions is important when applying for a position as to which document the employer is requesting. Resumes and CVs provide you an opportunity to "sell yourself" to your future employer. Use these tools to highlight your academic and career achievements. They are your future employer's "first impression of you."

TABLE 4-1

Sample Resume	
NAME:	JANE DOE
ADDRESS:	1111 MAIN STREET
	COLUMBUS, OH 44331
PHONE NUMBER:	
EMAIL ADDRESS:	
PROFESSIONAL SUMMARY	
SKILLS	
EXPERIENCE	
EDUCATION	
CERTIFICATION	

You may want to draft your own resume/CV or have it done professionally. Always proof your documents and utilize "spelling and grammar checks." There are many styles and formats available, so take a look at a few and decide which best represents you and the position you are seeking.

General Tips

Regardless of your choice of drafting your own document or having someone do it for you professionally, there are few things to keep in mind. These tips are for both resumes and CVs.

When listing your demographic information, it is important to give a phone number where you can talk privately if contacted. Future employers do not view using a current employer's phone number favorably. If you provide your cell phone number, be sure you will be able to take the call as well as have good phone reception. If providing an email address, be sure that it is professional in nature. You may want to establish a separate email account just for your job searching. The use of a current employer's email address is perceived the same as if you were

TABLE 4-2

Sample CV

CONTACT INFORMATION Name, address, phone number, email address	
EDUCATION (Chronological order, with university name, city and state, and degree awarded)	**Masters of Science in Nursing**—Post graduate—Adult-Gerontology Acute Care Nurse Practitioner. Kent State University, Kent, OH, December 2019. **Masters of Science in Nursing**—Clinical Nurse Specialist University of Pittsburgh, Pittsburgh, PA, May 2016. **Bachelors of Science in Nursing**—Youngstown State University, Youngstown, OH, May 2014.
LICENSURE & CERTIFICATIONS	**Registered Nurse Licensure (list all states licensed in)** State of Virginia, current through August 2020 State of Ohio, current through August 2021 **Certification** American Nurses Credentialing Center Acute Care Nurse Practitioner February 2010—present Certified Critical Care Nurse (CCRN) dates Certified Heart Failure Nurse (CHFN) dates Advanced Cardiac Life Support, current through August 2021 Basic Cardiac Life Support, current through August 2021
NP STUDENT CLINICAL EXPERIENCE 1. (ONLY if new graduate)	**Adult Acute Care** *Office-address dates* *Clinical Preceptor: Dr. and/or NP* Managed acute illnesses and chronic, complex, multi-system disease processes.

(Continued

TABLE 4-2

Sample CV *(Continued)*

	Counseled clients regarding smoking cessation, stress management, physical activity, and disease management.
	Cardiology
	Office-address dates
	Performed routine pacemaker and defibrillator management.
	Developed proficiency in the special needs of adults ages 60–100.
	Geriatric Medicine
	Skilled Nursing Center-address dates
	Objectives
	Geriatric Medicine
	Site and address dates
	Objectives
PROFESSIONAL EXPERIENCE	**(List in chronological order with month and year)**
	Graduate Student Teaching Instructor
	University of Pittsburgh, Pittsburgh, PA, 9/08-12/10/2016
	Graduate Teaching Assistant— Responsible for scoring of transtracheal patient questionnaires for NIH Clinical Trial.
	Staff Nurse, Clinical Nurse II
	Medical center employment dates
	Role: Provided tertiary care to a diverse population of critically ill cardiology and cardiac electrophysiology clients at a large academic affiliated medical center.
	Expertise in pacemaker and implantable cardiac defibrillator programming, cardiovascular exams.

(Continued)

TABLE 4-2

Sample CV *(Continued)*

Resource Nurse, Clinical Nurse II

Medical center employment dates

Adult Intensive Care Units

Cared for a variety of critically ill clients at a level one trauma center.

Cared for patients requiring mechanical ventilation, multiple drug infusions, post cardiac arrest, acute on chronic kidney disease.

Staff Nurse, Clinical Nurse II

Medical center employment dates

Medical Intensive Care/Pulmonary Medicine

Provided individualized care in the MICU at a large inner-city hospital.

Expertise in hemodynamic monitoring, pulmonary artery catheters, titrating drips, mechanical ventilation, and substance abuse management of the critically ill client.

Charge Nurse, Preceptor

Medical center employment dates

Cardiac Critical Care

Functioned as a charge nurse and staff nurse on a 16-bed cardiac step-down unit at a large teaching hospital in a primarily Arabic community.

Provided individualized care for coronary artery bypass graft and valve replacement surgical clients. Assumed responsibility for orienting and training student nurses and nurse orientees.

(Continued

TABLE 4-2

Sample CV *(Continued)*

	Assisted with staff scheduling and the introduction of clinical pathways.
	Expertise in cardiac arrhythmias, cardiac drips, pacemakers, and cardioversion.
AWARDS & HONORS	• Ruth Perkins Kuhn Award—outstanding graduate student in areas of research and education.
	• Sigma Theta Tau
ACADEMIC & PROFESSIONAL ACTIVITIES	• Sigma Theta Tau International Honor Society of Nursing, Member, dates of membership
	• American Association of Critical Care Nurses, Member, dates
VOLUNTEER COMMUNITY ACTIVITIES	• United Way Day of Caring, 2017
RESEARCH	Pilot study on "Effectiveness of Two Methods of Oral Suction in Intubated Patients." Funded in part by Bard Medical.
MANUSCRIPTS	**List any publications. Include columns in newsletters as well as journals, etc.**
PRESENTATIONS	• Annual AACN Chapter Meeting— Understanding Mechanical Ventilation
	Unit-based Education Committee— Presentation on Heart Failure
REFERENCES	**Please list specific pre-approved contact names, addresses, phone number, email addresses**

utilizing their phone number. It may lead the future employer to question your use of their future resources.

On your resume/CV in the subheading of licensure/certifications it is best not to list any certification, licenses, or DEA numbers. This will prevent someone from inadvertently having access to these numbers if your resume/CV was not in a secure location. It is appropriate to list the certifying organization and expiration dates. As a new NP you may be in the process of applying or waiting for results. If this is the case, it is acceptable to list "pending" beside the appropriate item. This section may be divided so that licensure is separate from certifications. It is appropriate to list your CPR, ACLS, PALS, and other such certifications with their expiration dates in this section.

Listing nurse practitioner student clinical experience is only appropriate for the first NP position post graduation. You will want to list each clinical rotation course and area separately. Identify the number of hours completed in each setting as well as any specific patient populations and the number of patients you saw on an average daily. If you performed any procedures identify them as well as if you performed them with assistance or independently. It is not necessary on your resume/CV to identify preceptors' names. You may want to support this information in your portfolio by utilizing the more detailed information available in Typhon or any other method you created for logging this information.

The Resume

Often the first impression a future employer has of you is from your resume. Remember the saying, "You only get one chance to make your first impression." Keeping this in mind, your resume is a significant snapshot of you. A resume (Table 4-1) is usually one to three pages in length. It follows a prescribed format and highlights your academic education, work history, and other relevant experiences in short, two- or three-sentence paragraphs or bullet items. Many large employers have computer software that scan resumes for keywords, and it is these computers that make the first "cut," weeding out the majority of the applicants before a human even sees the resume. Some tips on preparing your resume to avoid these pitfalls include using plain white paper. No need to spend the extra cash on formal stationary. Use basic print fonts of no less than 11 in styles such as Helvetica or Arial, and minimize or eliminate italics, bold face, and underline.[3] Be sure to explain all time gaps, if present, on the resume. Some legitimate reasons for time gaps are relocating, seeking employment, child or parental care responsibilities, or perhaps returning for further education. Sometimes these gaps are for legitimate reasons, but you don't want them to be a red flag. It is also not recommended to list references as "furnished upon request." It is best to provide names, addresses, and other contact information of individuals who you have discussed as future references. It is also helpful to the individuals you are requesting references from to provide them with some information about you as well as some of the specifics of the position you are applying for. By completing these few steps, you will be more likely to secure meaningful letters of reference.

You may underline in color the various section titles, or underline before and after the title. This enables areas to be emphasized appropriately. The resume is allowed to be less formal and more artistic in nature—still keeping it professional.

The Curriculum Vitae (CV)

The guidelines for a CV are similar to those for the resume regarding font style and size. Information included in a CV (Table 4-2) is as follows. Most CVs start with the individual's contact information. This is then followed by education and qualifications, work experience/employment history, as well as specific skills (computer, language, etc.). Education and work experience should be in chronological order with most recent being first. Be prepared in your interview to explain gaps in work experience/employment history as previously discussed. Tailor your CV for the position you are applying for. If you are applying for an educational role you will want to emphasize your educational experiences. If you are applying for an oncology position, emphasize your clinical rotations in this area. Do not use a "one-size-fits-all" for your CV. Learn to modify it for the position you are seeking. Make sure it is organized and has an uncluttered look. Keep subject headings in bold. Keep information in chronological order for ease of reading by the future employer. Keep explanations brief but informative.

ORGANIZING A PORTFOLIO

Portfolios give employers an in-depth look at your skills. They can get more information on a particular area of expertise—but keep in mind your resume must still be able to stand on its own. If you write a lackluster resume, no one will bother to look at your portfolio.[1] View your resume as a one-page, executive summary of yourself and your career. Make the reader want to know more about you.

One way to present all of your data in an organized manner is to create a portfolio. The easiest to complete is one that is in a notebook style where pages can be added or removed. Utilizing plastic sleeves to place the documents in prevents altering the status of the document as well as facilitates changing their order in the portfolio. According to Buppert[4] there are three reasons why an NP would want to compose a portfolio.

The first reason is to contain information regarding training related to the performance of specific procedures as well as the documentation of how many times that procedure was performed. This should be specific per procedure. You may want to include information from your syllabi as well as a procedure log identifying how many times you have performed the procedure proctored as well as independently. Although the institution you are being employed by will still perform their own focused review of your procedure performance it is important to supply this documentation that (1) you had educational content related to the procedure/skill and (2) you actually performed the procedure/skill as a student nurse practitioner.

Second, some states refer to scope of practice statements that have been adopted by national organizations that represent advanced practice nursing. If this is pertinent, you would want to include a copy of the document in your portfolio.

Finally, some nurse practitioners utilize their portfolio when interviewing in place of or in addition to their resume. Table 4-3 identifies an example of the items that might be included in your portfolio.[5] If you include your licenses, certifications, and other such documents in your portfolio, be sure they are copies and not the original documents. You may want to also include a copy of your state's Nurse Practice Act as well as a statement from your certifying body regarding the NP scope of practice.

Remember, this is your showcase.

TABLE 4-3

Portfolio Documents
Personal Statement—Objective or "Summary of Qualifications"   **Personal Documents—Education/Publications Certifications/Awards Licensure**
Portfolio Documents
Sample Cover Letter
Resume/CV
Letters of Reference
Special awards
Grade Transcripts
Graduation diploma(s)
NP Certification, DEA certificate (if available), RN/NP license, BLS, ACLS, PALS
Copy of Scholarly project/thesis/capstone- abstract
Publications
Interests-   • Copies of course outlines   • Appropriate Typhon data
Photo identification

SUMMARY

Your resume, CV, and portfolio are your first impression you make to your future employer. Make them stand out from the many others they will receive. What makes you unique? What makes you the one they want to hire? What specific item(s) on your resume will stand out and make you the one selected for an interview? Remember that they all are living documents. Be sure to keep them up-to-date. Make these documents specific for the position you are seeking. Developing the right foundation for these documents will enable you to continue to build upon them as your career advances.

References

1. University of Michigan School of Nursing. (2018, July 19). Retrieved from Emily Springfield Instructional Technology Designer. http://www-personal.umich.edu/~espring/resumes/

2. The Typhon Group Healthcare Solutions. http://www.typhongroup.com/npst.htm. Accessed September 2, 2020.

3. CyberCollege. http://www.cybercollege.com/510res.htm. Accessed September 2, 2020.

4. Buppert, C. (2014). *Nurse Practitioner's Business Practice and Legal Guide.* Sudbury: Jones & Bartlett Learning. ISBN 10: 1284050912.

5. Dillon, D. & Hoyson, P. (2013). From Graduation to Employment: A Guide for the New Nurse Practitioner. *The Journal for Nurse Practitioners*, 312–315.

5 The Interview

Your resume or CV got the attention you were aiming for. Congratulations! You've got an interview scheduled. Now what? The adage "only one chance to make your first impression" continues into the interview phase as well. There should be significant preparation and practice prior to the interview. The more prepared you are, the more likely your interview is to be successful. Your interview may be a phone interview, virtual or an in-person interview. The preparation should be similar for all.

PHONE INTERVIEWS

Some employers choose to do a phone or virtual interview first. This can be helpful to them in narrowing their pool of applicants. It also minimizes their expenses, particularly for out of town candidates. Clarify with the employer when the interview is scheduled—the date, time, and if they are calling you or you are calling them. For virtual interviews, confirm or secure the ZOOM or Webex access that will be used. Always get their name and phone number. Confirm all of these details; it's wise to even request a confirmation email. Be prepared and available to take your call 10 to 15 minutes prior to the scheduled time. It is best if you answer the call yourself and identify yourself when receiving the call. The advantage of a phone interview is that you may have some of your key materials directly in front of you to reference (i.e., job description, curriculum vitae). Have your questions ready and written down. It's a good idea to have a pen and paper close by to take notes during the interview. Sometimes it is hard to remember your question as you are waiting for the interviewer to finish their comment. Be sure when scheduling the phone/virtual interview that you are in a private location with good cell phone reception (if not using a landline). If your interview is to be virtual, many of the same considerations should be given. Be sure your background is not distracting and if choosing a computer background for the interview, make sure it is professional. Remember to silence your phone for the virtual interview and be in an inter-rupted location with good wifi access. Be sure this location is one with limited distractions or opportunities for disrup-tions (i.e., pets, children, other phones ringing). It is a good idea to prepare for the phone interview the same way as you would for the in person—not in your pajamas. You will want to practice this interview as well. Record yourself during your practice interview noting if you talk too fast or too slow, use a lot of "ums," or pause too many times. There is a fine balance between "dead air" and an appropriate pause for a response. You also don't want to rush into responding to a question just to end the silence. Sometimes you may need to request that the state-ment or question be restated so you can give your best response. Allow the interviewer to finish their sentence before you jump in with a response. It's a good idea to keep some drinking water available in case you develop a dry throat or a cough during the interview. Chewing gum or eating during the interview should be avoided. As the phone/virtual interview concludes, remem-ber to thank the interviewer for the opportunity and the time taken to interview you. You may even use this as an opportu-nity to request an in-person interview. Sending out a thank you email immediately after the call is also considered acceptable and recommended. It reiterates your genuine interest in the position. You can also utilize this email to briefly address any-thing you did not have an opportunity to discuss during your phone/virtual interview.

IN-PERSON/VIRTUAL INTERVIEWS

Preparing for the interview starts with the clothing you wear to investigating the business in which you have applied to. Be pre-pared! You want to dress for success. The first impression you will make at your interview is going to depend upon what you are wearing. This is not the time for "business casual." Even if the position you are applying for has scrubs for their daily attire, it is not an appropriate clothing choice for your interview. This means that if you are interviewing with at your current place of employment, today is the day to bring a change of clothing for the interview. Give your outfit some thought well before the interview. This allows for a trip to the dry cleaners or alterations if necessary.

For men, a suit and tie still make the best impression. Solid colors such as black, navy, or gray are always a positive. If the interview atmosphere is more causal, you can always remove the tie or jacket. It's not possible to produce a jacket and tie if the environment is more formal. Men choosing a long-sleeved shirt as opposed to short-sleeved, regardless of the season, is always preferred. The color of the dress shirt should be white or coordinated with the suit. A conservative tie coordinated with the suit is also a good match. This is not the time to display uniqueness or creativity with character ties—keep a solid color. Accompanying dress shoes with dark non-patterned socks complete the attire. Again, non-patterned dress socks are appropriate. Shoes traditionally match the color of your belt. This is a good time to go lightly on the cologne or aftershave. A small briefcase may be appropriate to complete your look to carry an extra copy of your CV or portfolio.

For women, if wearing a dress or skirt, keep the length of the dress/skirt appropriate for interviews. If your dress is sleeveless, a jacket or sweater is appropriate. The neckline should also be conservative. The hemline should remain appropriate when you are seated as well. For women the height of heels should be flat 3 inches. If wearing slacks, a suit or well-coordinated jacket and pants are appropriate. The slacks should be ankle length—not the time for capris or a dress shorts with a jacket. The dress shoes should be conservative in nature. If you are not comfortable in heels, it is better to wear a dress, flat footware than to struggle with the awkwardness in walking. Flip flops are never appropriate. Open-toed shoes are not preferred, but can be worn in the summer. This is not the time to show your individuality. Nails should be neatly trimmed or manicured. If wearing a nail polish, it should be neutral in color. Go lightly on perfume. Makeup should be appropriate for daytime. Jewelry should be limited to one ring, watch, and a small necklace. No visible piercings or tattoos. Hair should be styled in a professional manner. A small handbag or briefcase should complete your look.

There are always some general interviewing rules. Your cell phone should be turned off for the interview. Chewing gum is a "no." Do not present with a cup of coffee, soda, bottled water, or food in your hand as you walk in the door. Of course, always bring your best smile.

THE INTERVIEW—ETIQUETTE

No matter how many times you have been interviewed, it is always a great idea to practice in advance. This pertains to both phone and in-person/virtual interviews. You can ask a friend to help prepare and critique you. Practicing in advance will provide a degree of confidence when the actual event occurs. Record yourself using your iPhone or iPad. Observe for any excessive use of "uh and um" as well as your posture and mannerisms. Body language often says more than your spoken word. Sitting and standing straight are important. Leaning into a conversation displays interest. Slouching in your chair sends a variety of messages—none of which are positive. Keep in mind, do you look interested, bored, or nervous? Try to avoid closed body language—crossing arms in front of you. Avoid placing your hand on your chin/face. Try not to 'rock' the chair you are sitting it. These mannerisms can be distracting, particularly on a virtual interview. Knowing these characteristics in advance and being conscious of them can help minimize them on the actual interview day.

Be on time for your interview, even attempt to be 10 to 15 minutes early. If possible, do a test drive to the building if you are unfamiliar with the area. Do the test drive at the same time of day you will be going to you interview to account for traffic patterns, constructions, school sessions, or any other sources of delay. If you are unfamiliar with the location of the meeting place, find it in advance as well. Perhaps someone can meet you in the main lobby or building entrance if possible. Be courteous to the individual who greets you. Often this individual reports to the person you are meeting with and will share any pleasantries, positive or negative, that might occur.

The handshake is important. For men, this is usually not a difficult step. Keep in mind—not too hard and not to soft. Use one hand only. The two handshake is reserved for the politicians. Stand up when shaking hands—meet at their eye level. Eye contact shows recognition, confidence, and respect. Smile when you enter the room.

Smartphones—don't want to see it—don't want to hear it. This too shows respect of the interviewer's time. It shows the importance you feel of the individual and interview. Keep your phone in the silent mode or turned off. Keeping it in your purse or briefcase will limit your distraction.

Finally, always remember to send a personal, handwritten thank you note. Send a separate thank you note to each person you meet. They should be genuine and point out some specific event related to your encounter with them.[1]

COMMON INTERVIEW QUESTIONS

Keep in mind that interviews should be about 50:50. Fifty percent questions: fifty percent listening. All interviews are unique, but most will have some common questions. One question you should have prepared in advance is, "Why should we hire you?" This question may be presented in a variety of ways. You should have a couple of rehearsed answers ready to roll out. The employer is looking for what it is that you uniquely bring to the position. This question may be phrased as "What else should we know about you?" This is your opportunity to expound upon your unique characteristics. They are evaluating your communication skills and confidence. Be prepared to give examples of why these are unique to you. Emphasize your work and clinical experience. Only give positive statements.

The following are other examples of common interview questions:

- Why should I hire an NP?
- How many patients do you anticipate seeing in one day?
- What can you bring to this practice?
- What is your greatest job strength? Weakness?
- What is your scope of practice? (It's also a good idea to have a copy of this in your portfolio.)
- Where do you want to be in 5 years? 10 years? Looking at your short-term or long-term goals?
- What are your thoughts on working weekends and evenings? Being on call?[2]

It is a good idea to review the business's mission statement and philosophy. Look for how you fit into this model. You may be asked what you know about the company or the practice. Spend some time doing your homework on the company or practice. If you are not familiar with the location of the business, it might also be wise to look at a few key landmarks or some significant data on the community. Who are other members that you will be working with? If you are the first NP in this practice setting, be well prepared to discuss your scope of practice and the differences you bring versus the RN, PA, and/or physician in the group. Be familiar with the scope of practice in the state in which you are applying for employment. This information should be presented in a positive, informative, non-threatening manner.

What are your strengths? What is your confidence level? Avoid one-liners. Even if the question requires a yes or no response, think of how to expound on that.

What are your weaknesses? Don't be extremely negative about yourself. I get angry easily is better phrased as "I'm a perfectionist."

Tell me about a difficult experience and how you handled it. Don't go into lamenting about a prior position you had. No one wants to hear that.

How do you handle change? Give an example of how you have done this in your prior role as an RN or during your NP education.

How well do you work under pressure? What happens when you get stressed out—do you panic or methodically think about what's going on. Be prepared with a couple of good examples where you can demonstrate your ability to handle pressure.

How do you handle important decisions?

How do you handle conflicts? You may be asked to provide an example of how you resolved one in your practice setting.

Questions may be specialty specific. Tell me about your experiences with caring for patients who have chronic pain needs? What is your experience with medications for chronic pain management? Be familiar with the area in which you are applying and be prepared for these specialty-specific questions.

Thinking in advance and planning your response(s) will make you feel more confident during your interview process. Role-playing through some of the above scenarios will help you to appear confident and knowledgeable about your future position.

AGENDA

Hopefully you will be provided an agenda for your interview day. It should include who you are meeting with, their title, and time frame for the meeting. Becoming familiar with the individuals you will be interviewing with is important. Are you being interviewed by an NP or a physician or perhaps both? What is the reporting mechanism in the institution? Are you reporting to nursing, medicine, or both? These are important factors to look at when considering how your role may be implemented. Who do you report to immediately—another NP or a physician? What are the backgrounds of the individuals who are interviewing you? Try and find out a little about their educational and professional backgrounds. Sometimes you may find common-alities, such as attending the same university or working with a former employer.

Information about the individual(s) who you are interview-ing with can be found by performing a Google search of the indi-vidual's name, searching LinkedIn, or reviewing the employer's website. Utilizing LinkedIn, you can access information about things you may have in common with the interviewer. Remember if you can access information about them, they can access infor-mation about you. Review your social media websites and delete information that might be embarrassing or viewed as not favor-able. Google your own name and see what information presents itself. You can be sure your future employer has done this.

If you are relocating to a community that is new to you, research the area. It's a good idea to know a little of the commu-nity's history. What is the size of the facility you are applying to? Is the service you are looking to work is new or been in existence for a while. What is the community known for? Some employ-ers may provide you with a gift bag at your hotel featuring some of these unique features of their community (e.g., local cider, candy Cardinal [state bird], sports memorabilia). You may also explore housing opportunities and may have arrangements to meet with a realtor during your visit.

Becoming familiar with your interviewers and the com-munity show you have an interest in them and the area. These topics can be good conversation topics as well as show you are interested in this position and you did your homework.

ADDITIONAL THOUGHTS

The interview is also a time to explore specifics about the job description, orientation and orientation length, working hours, call time, vacation, and paid time off. Have an idea in mind prior to your interview of what your thoughts are on these items. Compile a list of questions that you would like answered about the position as well. Often at the end of the interview you will be given time to ask these unanswered questions.

Some new graduates are so happy to secure their first position that they overlook some of these important factors that can impact on their job satisfaction later. Often a disappointment to new graduates is that the first NP position is "like starting all over." You may be leaving an RN position with 4 weeks' vacation for a new NP position that offers 2 weeks. Your initial salary will be representative of a new NP and may not vary significantly from your experienced RN salary. Anticipating some of these changes in advance can limit your disappointment during your interview.

At the conclusion of the interview you often have your own thoughts on how the interviewing process went. It is normal to reflect and focus on the items you may have answered differently given another opportunity. Always try and summarize why you are the best candidate for the job. Restate your interest in the position. The interviewer may have left you with a positive feeling that you were likely to secure the position. They may even request names and contact information for references. Be sure to have this information readily available. Always be sure you have discussed your reference's willingness to provide information when contacted.

Sometimes there is a mutual decision at the end of the interview that it was not the position for you or you for it. Whatever the outcome, learn from the interviewing process and take those thoughts with you for future interviewing. Not everyone gets offered the first job they interview for and not everyone accepts the first position they are offered.

References

1. Post A. (2018, July 19). TED-ED—Put Those Smartphones Away: Great Tips for Making Your Job Interview Count. https://www.youtube.com/watch?v=NKBlWanXzGE. Accessed July 19, 2019.
2. Buppert, C. (2018). The Employed Nurse Practitioner. In C. Buppert, editor. *Nurse Practitioner's Business Practice and Legal Guide* (p. 340). 6th ed. Burlington, MA: Jones & Bartlett.

6
Employment Contracts

You're considering your first position of employment after graduation. You are so excited to finally be at this point, but you need to carefully consider the employment contract you may be offered. The future employer may have mentioned a contract. You may be uncertain as to whether one is needed or not. This is a different perspective than your first position as an RN. You may not be offered an employment contract if employed in a hospital system. What should you know or consider? Many states fall under "employment-at-will" provisions of law.[1] This means that an employee may be terminated "at will" or without cause. It also means that you may terminate your employment without cause. The advantage of a good employment contract is that it can protect you from this occurring. An employment contract also affords you the opportunity to discuss issues that may be problematic before they occur. The first thing to know and remember is the employment contract you will be presented with will be developed by your employer or their legal counsel. This means that the employment contract will most likely be written to favor the employer. You will want to carefully review it, and even consider seeking your own legal expert to advise you prior to signing. Seeking legal advice on your contract is not considered an act of "non-trust." The attorney you choose should be familiar with an NP's scope of practice and job description. If you are unable to locate an attorney specifically familiar with NPs, one who handles employment law or contract negotiations would be appropriate. Three important clauses in an employment contract are related to bonus formulas, restrictive covenants, and termination clauses.[2]

EMPLOYMENT CONTRACT VERSUS COLLABORATIVE PRACTICE AGREEMENT

Before we start discussing the employment contract, it is important to clarify the difference between an employment contract versus the collaborative practice agreement. Employment contracts are written (usually by the employer and reviewed by the NP who makes recommendations or suggests changes) and signed agreements between the NP and the employer.[3] Although not required, an employment contract is a legally binding agreement that is signed by both parties. An employment contract is different than and does not replace a collaborative practice agreement. Not all employers will require an employment contract. If you practice in a state that requires a collaborative practice agreement you will have the collaborative practice agreement in addition to your contract.

Collaborative practice agreements are required in states in which NPs cannot practice independently.[1] Collaborative practice agreements are also written and signed agreements between the NP and the collaborating physician(s). In states with Full Practice Authority, there is no requirement for a collaborative practice agreement. Therefore, not all states will require a collaborative practice agreement. Although some of the content of both agreements may be similar there are significant legal differences. Collaborative practice agreements are usually defined by the state and include items such as coverage in absence of physician, referrals, process for review of documentation, and a plan for emergency care. It is not uncommon for the state board of nursing to provide a sample collaborative practice agreement for reference on their websites. You do not need an attorney to create the collaborative agreement. These agreements can and should be modified by you to meet your specific employment requirements. The collaborative agreement is also valid for a predetermined time frame, requiring periodic review and renewal. If employed by a hospital system, they may require that you adopt their standardized collaborative agreement form. Again, modifications can be made to "right fit" the agreement to your practice setting.

Collaborative practice agreements and legal contracts may contain overlapping items. Both employee contracts and collaborative practice agreements are legally binding documents. If you are employed in a state that requires a collaborative practice agreement and are required by your employer to have a written contract, review both documents carefully so that they are in alignment with each other.

EMPLOYEE OR INDEPENDENT CONTRACTOR

While most NPs will be employees it is important to understand the differences in the types of employment. If you are an employee, the employer's responsibilities to you are only what are specified in the contract. The employer is responsible for deducting payroll and other taxes. As an independent contractor it is not uncommon for you to be responsible for your own payroll taxes, health benefits, and malpractice insurance. In some instance the Internal Revenue Service has ruled that an independent contractor is really an employee because of how the employee relationship is set up. In making this determination, the "IRS looks at 3 sets of factors—behavioral control, financial control, and type of relationship—that provide evidence of the degree of control and independence."[4] Independent contractors can be terminated for any reason, pursuant to the conditions of a contract between contractor and contractee.[5] You may be hired as an employee or an independent contractor. Be sure you are familiar with the differences and your responsibilities if you are employed as an independent contractor.

CONTRACT DETAILS

Terms of the contract include the date of initiation, termination and renewal clauses. The compensation portion of your package addresses salary, expenses, bonuses, health and retirement benefits, as well as billing and reimbursement issues.[1] While you may be tempted to focus on your salary, there are other details you will want to be sure you have specific information on. You will want to pay close attention to details related to your work schedule. Are you expected to be on call as part of your new position? If so, how often. Ask for a description of what an evening or weekend on call is like (i.e., how many patients, how many calls on an average, is there a back-up physician on call). Is your contract for 1 year, 2 years, or longer? Most contracts are for 1 year. Does the contract state you will see a patient every 20 minutes from day one of employment or do you gradually increase the number of patients you will be seeing as you become more familiar with the patients, the practice, and the medical record system? Even if you are an experienced NP, by changing your practice specialty you may want to reduce the number of patients you initially see until you are comfortable in your new practice environment. In some states (i.e., Vermont) an NP obtaining a subsequent certification in an additional role and population focus practice requires a specified number of transition hours in that new practice environment.[6] Being unable to fulfill the requirements of the contract can lead to termination. This is an important detail which should be clear to a new practitioner. Do you have support staff such as a medical assistant or an RN to assist you with delivery of patient care? These support staff are key in helping you achieve your required number of patient visits per day. These variable amounts are all negotiating points. All contracts for NPs should include a variety of topics of discussion (Table 6-1).

Benefits and Compensation

The employment contract will also outline your benefit package. Salary, health insurance, sick time, and disability insurance are just some of the benefits to consider. This is not meant to be an inclusive list.

Salary

There are various ways in which an NP can be paid for as an employee. You may be paid hourly or as a salaried employee. Let's examine the differences. An hourly salaried employee is simply

TABLE 6-1

Items to be Included in Nurse Practitioner Contract

Salary
- Bonuses
- Vacation benefit
- Sick leave
- Personal leave
- Continuing education allowance
- Professional membership

Insurance
- Malpractice
- Life
- Health
- Disability
- Unemployment
- Worker's compensation

Retirement plans
- 401(k) or similar retirement package

Communication devices

Transportation

being paid for every hour of their work. A salaried employee is paid a fixed amount usually based on an annual projection. You may also have your salary calculated on a percentage of billing. An average hourly rate for a new NP is $57.00/hour. The average salary for an NP is $110,094.[7] Be familiar with what the entry-level salaries are in your community and state. How often will you be paid? Possibilities include weekly, biweekly, or monthly. Will your salary be based on what is billed or for what is received? This is a salary that is based on your patient billing. Being paid for billing as "charged" is preferred to being paid for billing as "received" or what was collected. The amount charged is often higher than the amount that will be collected from the billing submitted. This percentage may also be added to a base salary. Collections fluctuate based on the insurance market in the area you are employed. This method is particularly of benefit for a new NP.

For most RNs the transition from an hourly to salaried-wage cannot be underestimated. In a salaried position there is an unwritten expectation that you will usually work more than your stated weekly hours. Usually you will have more flexibility with a schedule that is salaried. Your hourly rate breakdown is higher if you are salaried to allow for this additional time requirement. If you accepted a position where you are always working late, frustration will quickly develop as you feel you are working for free. There are weeks when you are salaried that you will work more than or less than a 40-hour workweek. NPs should have an estimate of what their value is. If you find that you are always working significantly more than 40 hours/week, you may want to reevaluate and renegotiate this particular aspect of your contract.

Bonuses

In your contract discussions you may be offered an opportunity for a bonus. This opportunity is also often a first for new NPs. Questions you will want to ask include will there be a sign-on bonus? If so, what are the specific details of this bonus? Are there other bonuses available? How are they determined? How and when will the bonus be paid out? Is there a payback on the sign-on bonus if you leave the practice prior to a pre-determined time frame? Bonus formulas are calculations to determine addition monies when certain criteria are met. Always be sure this information is in writing and delineated in your contract.

Productivity-based Bonuses

Bonus formulas can be productivity-based and can be offered in a setting that is a fee-for-service model. This formula looks at the number of patients you see in a predetermined time frame. Essentially, you are rewarded for being productive and seeing more patients. For a new NP this may be a difficult bonus to achieve as initially you will be learning the practice, the patient population, and require more time to see patients. Depending on your practice arrangement, you may be building your new patient practice and have smaller numbers until you become established in the practice and the community. For this reason, productivity bonuses may not be achievable until you are in the practice for longer than 1 year. This method is also difficult to implement in a capitated system. Capitated plans pay the provider a fixed amount of dollars for care delivered regardless of the number of patient visits. Be familiar with the common payer methods in your community.

Quality-based Bonuses

Quality-based bonuses are made based on meeting or exceeding quality-based standards that are predetermined by the various managed care plans. This model is a bit more difficult to track. Managed care companies may require the NP to have their own panel of patients and/or be designated as a primary care provider for that panel. There are managed care providers that do not allow an NP to be a primary care provider. Where this arrangement is not possible, the NP and physician work as a team and the quality-based bonus would be a shared bonus. Again, a bit more challenging for tracking.

Profit-based Bonuses

As you can see from the above descriptions, bonus formulas can be quite complex. There are also bonus formulas that are shared with employees based on profits and/or based on patient satisfaction. Details on how these bonuses are calculated should be outlined in the contract. Whichever bonus method is offered, be sure you understand the bonus structure completely. Often having examples of the different formulas can provide clarity and understanding. Profit-based formulas can represent quite complex accounting methods. Be sure you retain the right to negotiate to audit the business's financial records. You should have access to your billing and receipts. Is there a dispute resolution guideline in your standard care arrangement/ contract if there is a discrepancy?[2]

Vacation

For beginning NP positions 3 to 4 weeks per year is an average amount of paid vacation time.[8] This may be another tough "pill to swallow" for the experienced RN who is now transitioning to a new NP position. Years of experience with one employer are usually rewarded with a significant amount of vacation or paid time off (PTO). Many RNs who return to school for their NP certification are experienced RNs and have accrued many weeks of vacation time. How many weeks of vacation will you have and when you will be able to take them? Is there "paid time off" if you work beyond your set work week hours? This is sometimes referred to as "comp time." In some salaried positions, the NP can take the time worked "extra" in 1 week and deduct it from the next week's work hours. Some employers refer to vacation time as "paid time off." You may have a minimum of 3 to 4 weeks per year, but additional compensation for time worked beyond set work week hours, or accrued through on-call coverage, may add to this baseline time allotment.

Continuing Education Allowance

Continuing education reimbursement is also a benefit to be negotiated. What will your reimbursement be per year? Typical continuing education allowances range from $1000 to $4000 each year. The average allowance is around $1500/year.[9] Will there be additional paid meeting time or will you be using vacation/ personal time for meetings. This can and should be a negotiating point. Do your benefits include payment for your RN, NP, and DEA renewals as well as other certification renewals? Some employers insist that professional licensure renewal is bundle into your continuing education allowance. Do not underesti mate the expense of these items and what an advantage havin them as a benefit could be. Collectively these items could tota over $1000 in expenses for the NP if not a reimbursable benefi

Malpractice Insurance

Carrying malpractice insurance will probably be a new consid eration for the new NP. While a separate malpractice plan ma have been an option to consider while an RN, it is a must hav as an NP. Some of the questions to consider are as follows. Wi the malpractice insurance be paid for by the employer and wi you have your own policy or be part of the group's policy? NP often consider a separate malpractice policy, on their own, a well. This enables the NP to have his/her own attorney in th event the malpractice incident is with one of the other provider in the practice. Inquire about tail coverage in the event you ter minate or are terminated. This can be a major expense to pur chase if you change employers. It can also be a major expens if a claim occurs after you have terminated your employmer and didn't realize you would need to purchase tail insuranc coverage. Have a clear understanding of the type of malpractic plan you have (occurrence or claims made). Occurrence-base policies provide coverage when the act occurred. Claims-mad based policies require the policy to be in effect at the time th act occurred and at the time the claim was made. The tail cover age provides coverage, in this event, if the claim is made afte the policy was in effect. More specifics related to malpractic will be covered in Chapter 8.

Retirement Plans

You will also want to inquire about retirement benefits. Is ther a 401(k) or a 401(k) match? The employer may also offer pension-profit sharing plan. Prior to employment you shoul have a basic understanding of the different retirement options. There are many types of plans such as Individual Retirement Accounts (IRAs), Roth IRAs, and Roth 401(k), just to name a few. If a retirement plan is not part of your contract you should arrange on your own to meet with a financial planner to explore available retirement planning options. If your employer offers you a choice in the retirement plan you choose, you should also schedule to meet with the financial planner to determine which option is best suited for you.

HOSPITAL-BASED EMPLOYMENT

Benefits may not be as negotiable when you are employed by a healthcare setting. In these environments, there are more "standard" benefits that are offered to all NPs and unfortunately may be the same benefits offered to all employees, exclusive of employed physicians. It is important to know in advance what your negotiating points are. Time off may be more valuable to some NPs versus a higher starting salary. A schedule that is flexible may also be more attractive to some NPs.

TERMINATION CLAUSE

There should also be in the employment contract rationale(s) for termination. What are the specific circumstances in which you could be terminated? Not that one wants to think about this as you are just starting a new position, but not fulfilling your contract (i.e., not seeing the required number of patients) can be a just cause for termination. There will be other items delineated in the employment contract that can lead to termination. Some are fairly standard and may include loss or suspension of your NP or RN license, unprofessional or unethical conduct, civil or criminal charges, or insurance fraud or abuse. If you are terminated is there a "non-compete clause" or sometimes referred to as a "restrictive

covenant"? A non-compete clause usually limits your ability t
practice within a certain predetermined mile radius.

What are the circumstances in which **you could termi
nate** your employment contract? Are they outlined specifically
Would you be given a 30-day notice or immediate dismissal wit
pay? Some examples in which you would want to consider te
minating your employment contract would be physicians' los
of Medicare/Medicaid participation, physician having a civil c
criminal charge, the employer fails to uphold your employmer
contract (breach).

RESTRICTIVE COVENANTS

Restrictive covenants, also referred to as "non-compe
clauses," define what location you may work in after termina
tion. Some restrictive covenants may require the NP to relo
cate as it may limit his/her ability to seek employment withi
a 30-mile radius for a specified time frame (i.e., it may be u
to 2 years). For NPs who terminate employment with a restric
tive covenant, this may require geographically relocating i
order to continue practicing as an NP. This should be give
significant consideration before agreeing to a contract wit
a non-compete clause. Termination clauses should speci
the circumstances in which employment may be terminate
Employment may be terminated with or without cause. The
may also be timelines associated with the termination claus
(e.g., immediate, 30 days, etc.). Be sure you know and unde
stand the details and ramifications.[5]

PROFESSIONAL ISSUES

In addition to benefits and compensation you should al
have specific details regarding professional issues in yo

employment contract. Some examples of these items are as follows: How will the billing be performed on your behalf? What
services are available for billing of your services? How are you
billing—under your own provider number or the physician's
provider number? What is your access to the billing service?
Will you be seeing patients and the physician signing off on the
note that also includes their billing for the service? Will you be
able to bill under your own insurance numbers and do both
independent billing as well as incident-to-billing? What is the
process for promotion within the practice setting? How often
will you be evaluated—6 months initially and then yearly? Is
your performance appraisal in alignment with your contract
negotiations? Another professional issue can be your title, name
on the door, letterhead, iphone/ipad for business use and/or
business cards.

SUMMARY

The NP employment contract is a new experience for most NPs.
An employment contract needs to be reviewed carefully prior to
signing. Be sure you understand it in its entirety. Do not be made
to feel that seeking legal advice on the contract is showing distrust
in the new employer. In states that require collaborative practice
agreements, these agreements should be in alignment with your
contract and vice versa. An employment contract has been lik-
ened to a marriage or prenuptial agreement. Be sure both parties
understand the document and agree upon it. Both sides of the
contract need legal counsel. Contract termination has been lik-
ened to a divorce, and like all documentation, if it's not written it
can be denied. You want the employment contract to protect you.
Don't hesitate to ask clarifying questions and to seek appropriate
legal counsel. It is important to clarify all details of your employment contract as well as being sure that all the details are in your
contract before you sign on the dotted line.

References

1. Brown L.A. & Dolan C. (2016). Employment Contracting Basics for the Nurse Practitioner. *The Journal for Nurse Practitioners,* 12 (2) e45–e51.

2. Buppert, C. (2018). The Employed Nurse Practitioner. In C. Buppert, editor. *Nurse Practitioner's Business Practice and Legal Guide* (pp. 331–342). Burlington, MA: Jones & Bartlett Learning.

3. Sample Contract: Nurse Practitioners in Primary Care. https://www.napnapcareerguide.com. Accessed July 24, 2018.

4. Buppert, C. (2012). Should an NP Take a Position as an Independent Contractor? *Journal for Nurse Practitioners,* 8 (8) 657–658.

5. Buppert, C. (1997). Employment Agreements: Clauses That Can Change an NP's Life. *Nurse Practitioner,* August 22 (8) 108–109, 112, 117–119.

6. State Law Chart: Nurse Practitioner Practice Authority. (2017). American Medical Association Advocacy Resource Center.

7. Nurse Practitioner salary in the United States. https://www.salary.com/research/salary/benchmark/nurse-practitioner-salary.August2020. Accessed September 4, 2020.

8. Employment Negotiations. American Association of Nurse Practitioners. https://www.aanp.org/practice/business-practice-management. Accessed July 24, 2018.

9. 7 Things You Should Consider in a Nurse Practitioner Employment Contract MidlevelU. https://www.midlevelu.com/blog/7-things-you-should-consider-nurse-practitioner-employment-contract. 2012. Accessed September 17 2018.

7 Negotiating a Salary

Salary negotiation is often another first for the new NP. As a RN, for the most part, your salary was fixed with limited or no negotiation. Similar to discussing your contract, discussing your salary is another area that brings discomfort to all parties involved. This is an area that you should do some research in prior to your discussion. The American Association of Nurse Practitioners[1] website is an excellent source of downloadable information regarding employment considerations. Advance for NPs and PAs[2] also provides salary information collected through their annual survey as well as employment strategy information. In your new position you will be considered a generator of revenue. The NPs should always remain aware of how much revenue they generate in relation to the salary that is being requested. You also want to be aware of what your expenses to the practice will be as well. You want to be sure your expenses are worth the benefit. Or that at least your benefit to your employer outweighs your expenses.

Salaries vary depending on location in the country, specialty practice, and full or part-time position just to name a few. Being familiar with the salary structure in your community is important. You may have more of an ability to negotiate your salary in a private practice versus a hospital setting where the salaries may be preset. If the practice location you have chosen has never employed an NP, they may seek your input into salary recommendations. You should have knowledge on what are the usual and customary starting salaries for NPs in your community. Find out as well, what type of benefit packages others have been able to negotiate.

BASIC CONSIDERATIONS

When negotiating your salary, you will also want to consider the total compensation package that was negotiated in your employment contract, not just the salary. Practice expenses associated with your employment may range from 20% to 50%

depending on the practice size, and this amount will need to be adjusted from the revenue you generate.[3] Practice expenses include, but are not limited to, malpractice insurance, support staff for the NP, health insurance (e.g., vacation, sick leave, continuing education, office supplies).[4] A lower starting salary may be considered if you have a significant benefit package. A higher starting salary may be negotiated if the position offers limited or no benefits. Do not underestimate the value of your benefit package. Malpractice, disability, and health insurance are expensive if purchased on your own. Although you might not be worried about retirement now, retirement packages can have employee contributions that are from pretax dollars. These benefits should be taken advantage of if offered.

METHODS OF PAYMENT

In order to better determine your salary request, an understanding of the various methods of payment is helpful. Traditionally there are five methods of payment available.

A **straight salary** is a fixed amount to perform that is paid per the job description. This salary may also be paid as a fixed amount per day if the NP is working on a part-time basis. A straight salary is frequently what an NP is offered when employed in a hospital setting. Salaried positions are often higher than an hourly rate position as it is anticipated that the employee will be working more than 40 hours per week.

An **hourly rate** method of payment is what the NP was familiar with when working as an RN. You are paid hourly for your work. There is a certain figure that is agreed upon as an hourly rate. The NP is then paid that amount times the number of hours worked per pay cycle. If there is not a benefit package offered, the hourly rate can and should be increased.

A straight salary and hourly rate salary are the two methods most NPs are familiar with. They are also the most common salary arrangements. Physicians commonly use a productivity-based formula for salary negotiations. Two of these methods are percentage of net receipts and base salary plus percentage.

If you are paid based on the amount that you bill minus the account receivable and minus your portion of practice expenses, you are being paid based on a **percentage of net receipts**. If this is the payment method that is offered be sure it is for the amount billed (charged) and not the amount that will be collected (received). There is a significant monetary difference between these two methods. The amount collected is usually less than the amount billed for and will vary dependent upon the insurance carrier's reimbursement. In the amount collected payment version, this is a variable that you will not be able to change as the amounts are set by the insurance payors. In this instance it is important to find out what the payer mix is in your locale.

A **base salary plus percentage** guarantees you a base salary and provides additional income based on productivity. This method provides an incentive for the NP to make additional income. The drawback of this type of arrangement is that members in a group can become negatively competitive. It can also positively motivate individual providers to be more productive.[*] Be sure there is a clear explanation in your contract describing how this productivity bonus will be calculated.

HOW DO I KNOW HOW MUCH REVENUE I WILL GENERATE?

It is safe to say that as a new NP you will see fewer patients than you will see when you have gained some experience and comfort level in your new practice. Time will be needed to become comfortable with the support staff and the electronic medical record/documentation system, and in some situations, building your patient base. Think carefully about how many patients it will be reasonable for you to see in 1 day. Did you determine a set number in your employment contract? Take into consideration if the patients are existing patients being seen as a follow-visit, new patients, urgent patient visits, or some combination of the preceding. Remember in the beginning of your practice even follow up patients will be a new patient to you and may require additional time to be seen. There are usually different time intervals assigned to these visits as they vary in complexity as well. Different levels of reimbursement are also assigned to account for these factors. Even to an experienced provider this combination can impact on the volume of patients seen per day. Are all of the patients being seen in the same practice setting or will you be seeing patients in multiple locations on the same day. If you are seeing patients in a hospital setting and office setting (or multiple office settings) consider allowing travel time between the two practice sites. If you are traveling between practice sites are you being reimbursed for the travel expenses. If your travel between practice sites involves responding to emergency situations (i.e. birth and deliveries, care of neonates, or other emergency services) you should inquire with your automotive insurance carrier if additional coverage is required.

FEE-FOR-SERVICE

Initially you can roughly determine projections of revenue generation by determining the number of patients (both new and existing) you will see in 1 day and average the evaluation and management (E/M) codes (levels 2–5) for this daily average of patients, and multiply this amount by the reimbursed amount. This is the fee-for-service method.

An example would be that initially you see 10 patients per day. Assume for this example that they are all follow-up visits and will generate approximately $35.00/visit. You will generate $350.00/day. In actuality this daily amount will vary dependent on the code level and also the reimbursement per the insurance provider. In 6 months, or sooner, you may be seeing 20 patients per day ($700.00/day). You negotiated 2 weeks of vacation, 1 week of continuing education (CE), and 1 week of sick time. Based on the $700 per day you can calculate an annual revenue of $168,000/year. This amount will depend on the collection rate of the practice. Although this sounds awesome, this total amount is not all revenue. Subtract from this amount the 48% overhead expenses (rent, benefits, CE, etc.)[5] and the amount becomes $87,360. Initially you may require more physician consultation, which is estimated to be 15%. The revenue now becomes approximately $62,160. An additional deduction of 10% for employer profit leaves $45,360 in profit. These values will change as the values in the equation change (e.g., 3 weeks of vacation, etc.).[4]

ON-CALL TIME

Salary should also vary if there is an expectation to take call for the practice/service. You will need to determine what percent of the other providers' salaries in the practice are attributed to this activity. You would expect to receive a like percentage if you take call in rotation with other providers.[5] The frequency of your calls rotations (i.e. twice montly, quarterly) and the anticipated number of calls received during your rotation should also be taken into consideration. You will want to inquire as to the number of patients that are usually seen during a weekend call rotation as well as availability of a backup physician. After you have been on call, is the next scheduled work day a "day off" or will you be expected to work additional hours that week. Clarity now lessens disappointments later. As previously discussed, in Chapter 6, this is an item that should be outlined in your employment contract as well.

REVENUE IS NOT THE COMPLETE PICTURE

The total revenue generated does not tell the whole picture. By employing the NP, it enables the practice to see additional patients. If the NP practices in a setting with a surgeon, patients can still be seen if the physician is delayed in the operative setting. This enables new consults, in-patients, and discharges to continue seamlessly. Seeing patients on an urgent basis can reduce emergency room visits. Treating a patient urgently can also reduce hospitalizations (e.g., early heart failure assessment and management). These are not minor considerations. If the NP improves wait times for visits, patient satisfaction, and outcomes these are indirect benefits to the practice and can be rewarded in quality-based bonuses.

Improvement in patient satisfaction is significant for all employers, particularly hospitals where it impacts on Medicare reimbursement by 2% points.[6] The HCAHPS (Hospital Consumer Assessment of Healthcare Providers and Systems) was developed as a method of measuring patients' perceptions of their hospital experience. HCAHPS was implemented so a national standard for collecting and publicly reporting information about the patient experience of care could be made across hospitals locally, regionally, and nationally.

PERFORMANCE EVALUATION

During the interview process discussion should be held as to how and when your performance will be evaluated. One common method of measurement is the number of patients seen per specific time interval (i.e., month, quarter). Evaluation can also be made by the number and quality of procedures performed. Still others evaluate on revenue generated. Each employer has their own method or combination of methods for evaluating your performance. Knowing what you will be evaluated on helps you achieve these goals. If the practice does not have a performance evaluation method, this is an opportunity for you to develop a custom one with standards that match your practice.

SUMMARY

Salary negotiation is usually an unfamiliar territory for NPs. Research on some of the basics of negotiating is important. While the salary is not an insignificant factor, it has to be taken into consideration with several other variables. The salary may be reflective of the total benefit package. A strong benefit package may allow for a reduced annual salary. The cost of benefits cannot be minimized. The experience and expectations of the new NP also influence the salary. As you gain experience and increase the volume of patients being seen, you increase your value to the practice. Salary negotiation is like a dance with a new partner—often awkward in the beginning, but improves with time and expertise.

References

1. American Association of Nurse Practitioners. http://www.aanp.org. Accessed September 16, 2020.

2. 2018 Nursing Salary Guide. Advance Healthcare Network. elitecme.com/resource-center/nursing/2018-salary-survey-results/. Accessed September 16, 2020.

3. Dillon, D. & Hoyson P.M. (2014). Beginning Employment: A Guide for the New Nurse Practitioner. *The Journal for Nurse Practitioners*, 55–59.

4. Buppert, C. (2018). How to Negotiate a Reasonable Agreement. In C. Buppert, editor. *Nurse Practitioner's Business Practice and Legal Guide* (pp. 337–339). Burlington, MA: Jones & Bartlett Learning.

5. Employment Negotiations. American Association of Nurse Practitioners. https://www.aanp.org/practice/business-management. Accessed September 16, 2020.

6. Centers for Medicare and Medicaid Services. https://www.cms.gov. Accessed September 16, 2020.

8 Malpractice

Malpractice is word we don't want to hear. What exactly is malpractice? Negligence is the failure to follow the standard of care that any reasonable NP would provide under the same or similar circumstances. Malpractice occurs when a standard of care has not been followed and results in an injury. Determining malpractice determines if the injury was a result of the provider being negligent. Practicing following established societal guidelines and staying current in the literature of your area of specialization are ways to minimize the risk of malpractice. Common allegations against NPs were found to be "failure to diagnosis or delay in diagnosis, improper care and treatment, failure to refer patients to emergency care and improper prescribing or management of medications."[1]

All of us are concerned about malpractice. We promise to "do no harm" to our patients. Despite diligence and a variety of safety mechanisms that are built into our system, mistakes still happen. Medical errors are the third leading cause of death in the United States.[2] The annual list of the leading causes of death in the United States is compiled by the Centers for Disease Control and Prevention. The data is retrieved from death certificates. Death certificates have a major limitation of needing to assign an International Classification of Disease (ICD) code to the cause of death. Death certificates in the United States are used to compile national statistics. They have no facility for acknowledging medical error. The system for measuring national vital statistics should be revised to facilitate better understanding of deaths due to medical care. Appeals have been made to the CDC to revise the current system and expand the causes of death beyond diseases, morbid conditions and injuries.[3] ICD codes are the codes used for billing for services rendered. Until recently, there was no code for medical errors. The ICD classification of error, referred to as a misadventure diagnosis, has a separate set of ICD-10 diagnostic codes. The ICD 10 code is misadventures to patients during surgical and medical care. The codes range from Y62-Y69. The definition of misadventure is harm from or adverse reactions to medical

TABLE 8-1

Common Reasons for NP Litigation
Failure to diagnose or a missed diagnosis
Delay in diagnosing
Failure to treat
Medication errors—relating to improper prescribing or management
Failure to refer

Source: Data from Nurse Practitioner Malpractice Statistics.[1]

treatment. Descriptions of misadventures include adverse reactions to medical or drug contamination, foreign objects left in the body, drug dosage errors and blood misadventures. As previously stated, using established protocols, following societal guidelines, and listening to our patients are known to reduce the error factor. Knowing your scope of practice and staying within your scope of practice can also reduce the likelihood of litigation (Table 8-1).

Despite our necessary concern regarding malpractice for NPs, the incidence fortunately remains low for NPs. The American Association of Nurse Practitioners (AANP) fact sheet indicates that there are more than NPs licensed in the United States.[3] NP malpractice rates remain low with only 1.1% being named as a "primary defendant" in a malpractice case.[4] In a study conducted by a "large medical malpractice insurance company" the number of adverse incidents and claims involving NPs between January 2007 and December 2011 totaled 1800. Of those 1800, 200 were analyzed because of the amount paid by the insurance company. This was due to a judgment against the NP that was in excess of $10,000.00.[1] In this study it was determined that the average payment for the 200 closed claims was $221,852.00, which represented an increase of 19% for average payments made from a prior 10-year period. Ninety-six percent of the NPs for whom payments were made to the plaintiff in excess of $10,000.00 had individual policies (as opposed to policies issued to a medical practice or clinic).[1]

Unlike an RN position, the NP position requires you have malpractice insurance. This is no longer an option. Hospitals require you to have malpractice coverage as part of your credentialing process. Malpractice insurance will hopefully be offered as part of your benefit package. Even if malpractice insurance is part of your benefits, you may still want to consider a separate/ individual policy. There are mixed opinions on this philosophy of carrying a secondary malpractice policy. It is thought by some[5] that if the plaintiff attorney learns that an NP has a secondary policy, the NP will be named to obtain access to the policy. That secondary policy is considered another source of money for the plaintiff.[5]

If it is not part of your benefit package, you will need to purchase your own malpractice insurance. You should be prepared with some basic knowledge about malpractice policies when applying for a position. The price of malpractice policies varies depending on the type of policy, location of the practice, specific NP specialties, full and part-time status in addition to NPs who own their own practices.

SEPARATE OR A GROUP MALPRACTICE POLICY

If the malpractice policy is part of benefit package, is the plan separate or a group plan that includes other providers in the practice? The disadvantage of a group plan is that the plan is also defending your employer, which makes you at risk of not having your interests adequately represented in the event a claim is filed. This can occur if the same attorney represents two providers in the same practice. Having a separate malpractice policy enables you to have separate legal representation. This representation will assure your best interest is being considered. You may want to have your own malpractice insurance policy in addition to that provided by your employer. As discussed previously, there are differences in opinion on obtaining a second, separate malpractice insurance policy.[5]

NPs who consider working outside of their main place of employment, and/or "moonlighting," will need a separate malpractice policy. Each employer's malpractice only covers the NP while you are working in their employment.

MALPRACTICE COVERAGE

The type of malpractice offered will either be claims made or occurrence. Most hospital employers offer a claims made insurance.[6] NPs should ask for a copy of the malpractice policy for review prior to beginning employment.

Standard malpractice coverage is $1 million per event and $3 million maximum. This means that the maximum payable on any one claim is $1million and the number of claims that could be paid as a total annual aggregate is $3 million. The maximum the insurance carrier will pay in 1 year is $3 million. It is important to know if the legal costs are included within the liability limits. What does this mean? An example of this would be a litigation with damages of $1 million. Legal expenses in this situation could be $250,000. This means the total damages paid would be $750,000.[7] If this was the incident, the NP would be left paying the remaining amount. This payment may include your personal assets. The standard $1/$3 million malpractice coverage policy is what is usually required by hospitals during the credentialing process. High-risk practices may be required to have a higher level of coverage (i.e., $2/$6 million). Examples of high-risk practices may include nurse midwifery, critical care, and neonatal care.

With the above being said, you should not just go out and purchase a higher malpractice coverage plan. Your malpractice coverage amounts should be consistent with your employer's or other providers in the practice. Do not accept a plan that insures you for more than the other providers. The term "suing deep pockets" refers to suing the individual/employer who offers the most to gain from financially. Investigate the coverage of the other providers.

CLAIMS MADE VERSUS OCCURRENCE INSURANCE

Two types of malpractice policies exist—claims made and occurrence.[6] Claims made policies cover incidents that occur during the time the policy is active—in other words, while you are employed by that employer. Should you decide to change employers or to retire in the future, with a claims made policy, you will need to purchase what is called a "tail" policy. Tail coverage will provide legal protection in the event that you are sued after you terminate your employment. Litigation can occur several years after an event. The purchase of a "tail policy extension" of your policy can be quite expensive (i.e., $20,000). Even though tail coverage is expensive, so is a malpractice case that occurs after you have left that employer. You don't want to find yourself without coverage in that circumstance. Purchasing a tail policy extension will provide you peace of mind. The idea of a tail policy is usually new to NPs and can be overlooked when decisions are made to change employers. Some employers will cover the cost of a tail policy while in other instances, the NP bares the entire cost.

Occurrence insurance covers any incident that occurred while you were insured. It does not matter if the claim is filed after you have left that employer as the coverage was in effect at the time of the occurrence. If you are given the choice by your employer or are purchasing your own insurance, choose an occurrence malpractice policy. With an occurrence-based policy, there is not a requirement for tail coverage when employment is terminated. These policies may be more expensive, but they are worth the expense. Calculate the cost of the occurrence insurance versus the cost of tail coverage when making this decision.

How do you pick a malpractice insurance carrier? Know the financial status of your insurance carrier. There have been instances where the insurance carrier was out of business at the time of a claim filing. Look up the financial rating of the carrier in advance. It is not recommended to accept anything less than an A+ rating.[7] Hospital credentialing evaluates the malpractice carrier as well and may not accept companies with less than an A+ rating. Hospitals may also not accept carriers that are located outside of the United States. If you are selecting your own malpractice carrier, it is advisable that you check with your employer and the hospital credentialing requirements to see if the carrier is acceptable to their criteria before you make your purchase.

WHAT IF YOU ARE SUED?

Sometimes you are suspicious about a potential litigation and at times you are certain that an event has occurred that will most certainly end in litigation. Some states (e.g., Ohio) have what is called a "180-day letter" or a "letter of no intent." This letter is designed to allow the patient an additional 6 months added to their 1-year statute of limitations to file their claim. If the 180-day letter is received within the 1-year time frame it "gives to the person who is the subject of the claim written notice that the claimant is considering bringing an action upon that claim."[8] "This statute was enacted in order to decrease the likelihood of frivolous medical malpractice actions by allowing the putative plaintiffs additional time to investigate the claims if brought to the attorney's attention moments before the expiration of the one-year statute of limitation," *Marshall v. Ortega, 87* Ohio St. 3d 522, 523 (2000).[8]

If you are in receipt of a 180-day letter or a letter notifying you of a litigation, contact your malpractice carrier and notify them of the lawsuit. They will request a copy of the letter for review as well. If the litigation is against the group you are practicing with, request your own legal representation. It is important that you do not discuss the potential lawsuit with anyone, especially the plaintiff (patient) or their legal representation. You will of course review the patient's record to refresh your memory of the patient and the alleged incident. Do not alter the record after being notified of the litigation charge. Your attorney will advise you on the subsequent steps in the process.

- He/she will review the patient's record as well.
- You will meet with your attorney to review and discuss the case.
- A deposition—a pretrial information gathering session—can be performed as part of the preparation for the trial. "What you say during the deposition can lock you into what you may say at the trial."[9]
- Your attorney will advise you as to whether to "settle" the case. Careful consideration must be given when agreeing to a settlement as this information is reported to the National Practitioner Database and remains their indefinitely.

NATIONAL PRACTITIONER DATA BANK

Established in 1986 under the Health Care Quality Improvement Act, the National Practitioner Data Bank's (NPDB) mission is to improve the healthcare quality, protect the public, and reduce healthcare fraud and abuse in the United States.[10] The NPDB is a web-based repository of malpractice claims and adverse actions reported by hospitals, state licensing boards, and other such organizations. Insurance carriers are required to report all damage awards to the NPDB. This is the reason to carefully considering a settlement in a litigation. Hospitals are required to inquire into the NPDB with your initial credentialing and every 2 years for renewal of clinical privileges. The information in the NPDB remains there indefinitely. Providers can submit statements to the database on their version of the incident. These statements are listed as addendums with the case information. The NPDB was designed to protect the public from dangerous providers, which include physicians, dentists, NPs, and other healthcare providers, who may relocate in an attempt to keep their malpractice claims concealed. The NPDB cannot be accessed by the general public.[10]

A study analyzing malpractice claims between 2001 and 2007 that were reported to the NPDB showed that 37% of physicians and 3.1% of physician assistants were required to pay damages for malpractice claims filed by patients. During that same time period only 1.5% of NPs had to pay damages.[11] The rate for NPs paying damages from 2007 to 2016 rose only 0.6%.[12] These percentages are anticipated to increase with the increasing number of NPs practicing as well as the increased complexity of care being provided by NPs.

As part of the hospital credentialing process, the NPDB will be queried assessing for any entries on behalf of the NP. There are also questions on the "application for privileges form" that the NP must respond to that addresses a history of being involved in a litigation and malpractice payments. If a response is positive to these questions, often a separate form must be completed outlining the specifics of the litigation including amounts awarded. If there are more than one litigations to report, they are reported on separate forms.

Information in the NPDB is there indefinitely. This is the reason why awarding of a settlement is a careful and significant decision that should not be taken lightly. The NP may make an addendum to the date reported in the NPDB if they feel it will add clarity to the report.

STATE BOARD OF NURSING

If an NP is reported to the NPDB, the NPDB in turn reports this information to the NP's state board of nursing state BON. The state BON granted your license and has the ability to revoke your license or impose a disciplinary action. When the state BON receives notification from the NPDB, it then makes a determination whether to investigate the NP and pursue disciplinary actions. This is done in cases where the BON believes there was gross negligence performed by the NP.[13] If the judge in the malpractice case deems there was malpractice, they may report that information directly to the state BON.

This reporting then triggers the disciplinary process by the state BON.

- The NP will be notified via a letter that they are being investigated and to contact the state BON to arrange a meeting.

- The NP will meet with an investigator that will review the records or documentation of the care provided that is in question. The NP will be given an opportunity to provide an explanation to the documented care provided. The investigator gathers their information from a variety of sources including, but not limited to, colleagues, patients, administrators, and auditors.

- After a careful, thorough review of the documentation and interviews, the investigator will determine if the disciplinary process will proceed or if a hearing will be recommended.

- In the event a hearing, or trial, is recommended, the NP should have legal counsel present. The state BON will have a state attorney present.

- The NP may be given the option of a prehearing settlement conference. The NP, their attorney, a hearing officer or board member will be present at this conference. A recommendation from this prehearing settlement conference will be made to the state BON. The possible options are that the state BON could drop the matter or proceed with a discipline of the NP. The discipline may be probation, suspension, or revocation of a license.[13]

Remember that the role of the state BON is to protect consumers. Any disciplinary actions are public information and therefore accessible to the public. Often these disciplinary actions are reported in the bulletin that the state BON mails to their nursing audience.

There are also queries on the credentialing application if your license has ever been suspended or revoked. These must always be responded to with a yes, even if your license has been reinstated.

SUMMARY

The idea of malpractice insurance will most likely be new to most NPs. Understanding what type of coverage is available will enable you to make more informed decisions. Coverage of your malpractice insurance by your employer can be a great benefit. Questions to ask about the malpractice coverage include: Is the policy a claims made or occurrence? Is it the same policy as other members of the practice? and Are the coverage amounts the same as other members in the group (i.e., 1/3 million)? Some careful consideration should be given as to whether you purchase your own individual malpractice coverage in addition to the coverage provided by your employer. If you have a claims made policy, inquire about the cost coverage for tail insurance as well as will your employer cover this cost or will it be your expense in the event that you change employers.

In the event of a litigation, practices may become fractionated. Even consulting relationships can be stressed. The NP may find themselves alone to face the claim.[5] If your contract has an arbitration clause (or alternative dispute clause), any disagreement will be settled out of court. According to Brown and Dolan[6] this is basically a promise not to sue in court, but rather to file any claim(s), including contract disputes, through mediation/arbitration divisions of the alternative dispute section.

Staying within your scope of practice as defined by you state nurse practice act and staying current in your area of specialization are two ways of reducing your likelihood of a malpractice event occurring.[14] Being named in a lawsuit is emotionally devastating even if you are dismissed. The entire process may last a year or more from your initial notification letter. This can be a draining and stressful time. It can be a distraction while you are continuing to practice. If you are found liable, the consequences can be professionally devastating. Remember two things: (1) the number of NPs who are sued is small, with only 1% being named as a primary defendant in a malpractice case, and (2) patients who perceive their NPs as competent, compassionate, and courteous are less likely to be sued.[5] Keep these thoughts with you as well as the other recommendations to reduce your likelihood of litigation that were discussed previously.

References

1. Nurse Practitioner Malpractice Statistics. https://www.medicalmalpracticelawyers.com/blog/nurse-practitioner-malpractice/. Accessed September 16, 2020.

2. Medical Error: The Third Leading Cause of Death in the U.S. *BJM* 2016;353:i2139. https://doi.org/BJM.com. Accessed September 16, 2020.

3. Sipherd R (2018). The third-leading cause of death in the US most doctors don't want you to know about. Modern Medicine. CNBC.com/2018/02/22/medical-errors-third-leading-cause-of-death-in-America. Accessed September 16, 2020.

4. ICD 10 Data. icd10data.com/ICD10CM/Codes/V00-Y99/Y62-Y69. Accessed September 16, 2020.

5. American Association of Nurse Practitioners. (2018). NP Fact Sheet. https://www.aanp.org/all-about-nps/np-fact-sheet. Accessed September 16, 2020.

6. 2018 AANP National Nurse Practitioner Sample Survey. American Association of Nurse Practitioners. (2016). NP Fact Sheet. https://www.aanp.org/all-about-nps/np-fact-sheet. Accessed September 16, 2020.

7. Balestra M. & Thompsen A. (2014). Should Nurse Practitioners Who Are Covered by a Large Groups Malpractice Plan Also Maintain Their Own Malpractice Coverage? *The Journal for Nurse Practitioners,* 10 (10) 644–645.

8. Brown L.A. & Dolan C. (2016). Employment Contracting Basics for the Nurse Practitioner. *The Journal for Nurse Practitioners,* 12 (2) e45–e51.

9. Don't Make These Mistakes When Buying Your Malpractice Insurance. CMF Group. npjobs.com/malpractice/buying.mistakes.shtml. Accessed September 16, 2020.

10. Drafting the 180-day Letter in Ohio. https://www.smlegal.com. Accessed September 16, 2020.

11. Buppert, C. (2018). *Negligence and Malpractice in Nurse Practitioner's Business Practice and Legal Guide* (p. 284). Burlington, MA: Jones & Bartlett Learning, LLC.

12. National Practitioner Data Bank. https://npdb-hipdb.com. Accessed September 16, 2020.

13. Buppert C. (2014, April 1). What Happens When an Advanced Practice Nurse Is Sued? *Medscape.* Accessed September 16, 2020.

14. Nurse Practitioners and Professional Negligence Lawsuits. (2017, March 1). CPH & Associates. https://www.cphins.com/nurse-practitioners-and-professional-negligence-lawsuits/. Accessed September 16, 2020.

15. Buppert, C. (2018). *Risk Management in Nurse Practitioner's Business Practice and Legal Guide* (p. 300). Burlington, MA: Jones & Bartlett Learning, LLC.

16. Ulman J. (2015). How Often Are Nurse Practitioners Sued? nurse-practitioners-and-physician-assistants.advanceweb.com/Columns/Legal-Issues?How-often-are-nurse-practitioners-sued.aspx. Accessed September 16, 2020.

9

Insurance
Credentialing

In your new role as an NP you have the additional responsibility of providing patient services and generating revenue from those services. After the service has been provided, you will need to bill for that service and then submit that bill to the appropriate insurance carrier in order to be reimbursed. Part of the ability to generate revenue is being credentialed by the individual insurance carriers.

The credentialing process must be completed for you to be able to bill and receive payment for your services. In order to complete the insurance credentialing applications, you must be a graduate of a NP program. The NP program can be a master's, post-master's, or Doctorate of Nursing Practice (DNP) degree. Next you must successfully pass your national certification exam as well as be licensed in your respective state. You will also need to be employed as an NP. A practice address is necessary as this where the reimbursement funds will be submitted to.

If you are employed in a hospital setting, the insurance enrollment and training process, or the credentialing process, may be considered part of your on-boarding procedure. If you are employed in a private practice setting, frequently this credentialing process is performed by the practice/office manager. Most of the insurance or third-party applications are available online. Applying for third-party reimbursement may take weeks to months to complete before you are on the multiple provider panels. Attention to detail in completing the applications is essential to avoid delays in the credentialing process. Even if you are not the individual required to complete these applications, being familiar with them is important. Providing the practice manager, or designated individual, your curriculum vitae will assist them in performing the insurance credentialing process. The insurance credentialing process is often confusing for NPs. Becoming familiar with this process enables you to provide informed follow up if needed, as well as making sure you are a provider on all of the appropriate plans.

NATIONAL PROVIDER IDENTIFIER (NPI)

The first step in the insurance credentialing process is completing the application for an NPI number. The NPI number is a unique 10-digit number used to identify healthcare providers. The Health Insurance Portability and Accountability Act (HIPPA) of 1996 mandated a standard set of unique identifiers for health-care providers and healthcare plans. The actual implementation of the application process began in May 2005.[1] The purpose of the NPI number was to improve efficiency and effectiveness of the electronic transfer for health information.[1] The implementation of the NPI number was also intended to reduce costs as it was developed to streamline the electronic claims processes for providers. Centers for Medicare and Medicaid Services (CMS) developed the National Plan and Provider Enumeration System (NPPES) to assign these unique identifiers.

To be eligible to apply for an NPI number for the first time, NPs must be graduates of master's, post-master's, or DNP program, be nationally certified, and recognized in their states as NPs.[2] Each provider has their own unique NPI number that will be different from their practice's NPI number. The NPI number is applied for through the CMS National Plan and Provider Enumeration System. Although this number is applied for through CMS, the NPI number is used on all health insurance plans both private and public. The website for this application is https://www.nppes.cms.hhs.gov/. Application for this number should be completed first as all other third-party reimbursement applications will require your NPI number. Per the website, the online application will take approximately 20 minutes to complete (Table 9-1).[1]

There are other situations in which your NPI number will be utilized or required. Your NPI number must also be present on all prescriptions that you issue as well.[3] Pharmacists will contact you if the NPI number is not on your submitted

TABLE 9-1

National Provider Identifier
Date of birth
Social Security Number
State nursing license (Certificate of Authority)
Practice addresses, fax, and phone numbers

prescriptions. NPI numbers are also utilized on orders for durable medical equipment (DME).

Reimbursement is provided through six major categories of third-party payers. Each of the third-party payers requires separate applications.

- Medicare
- Medicaid
- Indemnity insurance companies
- Managed care organizations (MCOs)
- Businesses that contract for certain services
- Affordable Care Act—Obamacare

MEDICARE

Medicare coverage is the federal health insurance program for individuals age 65 or older, under 65 with certain disabilities, and for individuals any age with end-stage renal disease.[4] There are four parts to the Medicare program: Part A, B, C, and D.

Part A is what is commonly known as the hospital insurance. Part A coverage covers inpatient care which includes critical access hospitals and skilled nursing facilities (not custodial or long-term care). Part A also covers hospice care and some home healthcare. In order to be eligible for these benefits, beneficiaries must meet certain eligibility conditions. Medicare is paid for through employee's payroll taxes. Because a spouse may have already paid for Medicare Part A through their payroll taxes, most people do not pay a premium for Part A.[5]

Part B is for the medical insurance coverage. Part B is for the coverage for your doctor's services and outpatient care. In addition, it can cover some of the medical services that Part A does not cover. This may include services such as physical and occupational therapists and some home healthcare.[5]

Part C is for the Medical Advantage Plans that are the private insurance option for covering of hospital and medical costs. Part C was created out of the Balanced Budget Act (BBA) of 1997.[6] Medicare Part C provides Medicare beneficiaries the option to receive the Medicare benefits through private health insurance plans, instead of through the original Medicare Part A and B. The plans offered under Medicare Part C may include coverage for additional benefits such as prescription coverage or dental and vision coverage. Medicare Advantage enrollees pay a premium for Part B. The premium for Part B averages $130/month in 2018, plus the premium for their Medicare Advantage Plan.[7]

Prescription medication coverage is provided in Part D. Medicare Part D is available to anyone who is eligible for Medicare. To receive Medicare prescription drug coverage, individuals must join a plan approved by Medicare that offers Medicare drug coverage. Most individuals pay a monthly premium for Medicare Part D.[5]

Medicare Provider Enrollment

Effective with the passage of the Balanced Budget Act of 1997 by the Clinton administration,[6] all NPs, clinical nurse specialists, and physician assistants are eligible to bill for Medicare.[2] The requirement for their own billing number enabled these advanced practice nurses to bill for Medicare services. Prior to 1997 NPs did not receive reimbursement for their services unless they were provided in a rural/underserved area. The passage of the Balanced Budget Act was a huge step forward for NP advancement and recognition.

The Medicare paper application is CMS-855 855I. The form is available on the Center for Medicare and Medicaid (CMS) website at https://www.cms.gov/Medicare/CMS-forms/CMS-Forms-List.html.[5] The Internet application is a faster application process than the paper application. The website states that the enrollment is an average of 45 to 60 days when completed online. The Provider Enrollment, Chain, and Ownership System (PECOS) allows a method that is easy to check and update the status of your Medicare application. To enroll, you will need your NPI number and password.[8] There is a complete checklist on the PECOS website that outlines the information that you will need to complete an enrollment application (Table 9-2).[8] Utilizing this checklist will save you time as you can have all of your source documentation ready in advance which will expedite this application completion process. The PECOS website allows providers to run simple search queries to retrieve and view the status of their PECOS application as well.[5]

Some patients enrolled in Medicare are enrolled in MCOs as well. Medicare Part C refers to this plan coverage.

Keep in mind that typed forms are easier for Medicare to process, but the most efficient method for submitting your enrollment application is to use the Internet-based PECOS.[8] PECOS guides you through the enrollment application so you only supply information relevant to your application. PECOS also reduces the need for follow-up because of incomplete applications. Using Internet-based PECOS results in a more accurate application and saves you time and administrative costs.

Medicare claims are electronically submitted on a form called CMS-1500. Specific patient information is required on each form in addition to the specific diagnosis code (ICD), the procedure code (CPT), the charge, and the NP's NPI number. If the patient is enrolled in a MCO there are specific instructions for this submission which are discussed in the MCO section of this chapter.

TABLE 9-2

Before You Start: A Checklist for Individual Physician and Non-physician Practitioners Using PECOS

Below is a checklist of information that will be needed to complete enrollments via Internet-based PECOS:

✓ An active National Provider Identifier (NPI)

✓ National Plan and Provider Enumeration System (NPPES) User ID and password. Internet-based PECOS can be accessed with the same User ID and password that a physician or non physician practitioner uses for NPPES.
  ○ For help in establishing an NPPES User ID and password or assistance in changing an NPPES password, contact the NPI Enumerator at 1-800-465-3203 or send an e-mail to customerservice@npienumerator.com.

✓ Personal identifying information. This includes:
  ○ Legal name on file with the Social Security Administration
  ○ Date of birth
  ○ Social Security Number

✓ Schooling information. This includes:
  ○ Name of school
  ○ Graduation year

✓ Professional license information. This includes:
  ○ Medical license number
  ○ Original effective date
  ○ Renewal date
  ○ State where issued

✓ Certification information. This includes:
  ○ Certification number
  ○ Original effective date
  ○ Renewal date
  ○ State where issued

✓ Specialty/secondary specialty information

✓ Drug Enforcement Agency (DEA) number

(Continued)

TABLE 9-2

Before You Start: A Checklist for Individual Physician and Non-physician Practitioners Using PECOS *(Continued)*

✓ If applicable, information regarding any final adverse actions. A final adverse action includes:
  ○ Medicare-imposed revocation of any Medicare billing privileges;
  ○ Suspension or revocation of a license to provide healthcare by any State licensing authority;
  ○ Revocation or suspension by an accreditation organization;
  ○ A conviction of a Federal or State felony offense (as defined in 42 CFR 424.535(a)(3)(A)(i)) within the last 10 years preceding enrollment, revalidation, or re-enrollment; or
  ○ An exclusion or debarment from participation in a Federal or State health care program.

✓ Practice location information. This information includes:
  ○ Practitioner's medical practice location
  ○ Special Payment Information
  ○ Medical Record Storage Information
  ○ Billing Agency Information (if applicable)
  ○ Any Federal, State, and/or local (city/county) professional licenses, certifications and/or registrations specifically required to operate as a healthcare physician or non physician practitioner.

✓ Electronic Funds Transfer documentation—mechanism by which providers and suppliers receive Medicare Part A and Part B payments directly into a designated bank account.

cms.gov/Medicare/CMS-Forms/CMS-Forms/Downloads/cms855i.pdf

Source: Medicare Provider Enrollment (PECOS), U.S. Department of Health and Human Services. https://pecos.cms.hhs.gov/providers/index.html.

MEDICAID

Medicaid is a joint federal and state program that was designed to help individuals with limited income and resources with medical costs. States are not required to participate in Medicaid.

Medicaid also offers benefits not normally covered by Medicare, such as nursing homes and personal care services. The Medicaid program is for individuals of all ages whose income and resources are insufficient to pay for healthcare.[9] Medicaid is also for mothers and children who qualify on the basis of poverty and for adults who are disabled for the short term (1 year or less) and who qualify on the basis of poverty.[10]

Medicaid Provider Enrollment

There is a separate application to become a Medicaid provider. The Federal government has given most of the rule making and administrative duties for Medicaid to the individual states, and, in most situations, state law controls Medicaid activities.[9] This means that each state has its own individual Medicaid application. The applications are web-based. You apply through the individual state Medicaid agency. Requesting an application as an NP is done through the provider relations department.

Medicaid billing is also done electronically on the CMS-1500 form. The same patient identification information, ICD, CPT, and the NP's NPI number are required. If the patient is enrolled in an MCO there are specific instructions for this submission which are discussed in the MCO section of this chapter.

INDEMNITY INSURERS

An indemnity insurer is an insurance company that does not deliver healthcare, but pays for the medical care of those insured. Healthcare providers are paid on a per-visit or per-procedure basis in this model. Indemnity insured plans are frequently referred to as "fee-for-service" plans.[11] When an NP requests payment from an indemnity insurer the claim is submitted directly to the insurance company.

Indemnity plans do not require the patient to select a specific provider or to choose a specific primary care provider.

Unlike traditional plans where patients are required to see providers or facilities on a predetermined panel, indemnity plans afford the patients the freedom to choose their providers and hospitals. Patients who utilize these plans may pay for their services "up front" and then submit a claim for reimbursement. It is not uncommon for patients using an indemnity plan to pay an annual deductible before the insurer begins to pay for their claims. Similar to other health insurance policies, a fee-for-service policy requires a payment of deductibles and co-payments for the medical services.

Indemnity Insurer Provider Enrollment

Applying for an application for an indemnity insured plan requires calling the company to inquire whether a provider credentialing number is required. If so, you will need to apply and complete the required application. If no provider credentialing number is required, you may submit a CMS-1500 form to the specific company to bill for the services rendered.[10]

MANAGED CARE ORGANIZATIONS

MCOs are insurers that provide healthcare services as well as payment for those services. A health maintenance organization (HMO) is a prepaid form of an MCO. HMOs provide health benefits and financing with delivery of health services to its subscribers. Unlike the indemnity insurer plan, in MCOs the primary care provider has full responsibility for direction of the patient's care. More recently the term "medical home" has been coined to include these primary care responsibilities as well as providing preventative care, care coordination, and achieving positive care outcomes. Providers who work in this model may see additional reimbursement for achievement of these outcome measures. NPs have been gaining increased acceptance into MCO provider panels. When the NP is accepted into the MCO's provider panel they are designated as a primary care provider.

TABLE 9-3

MCO Panel Provider Membership

- Designation as a primary care provider
- Contract for providing care
- Credentialing application
- Directory listing
- Reimbursement

Provider panel membership includes several other responsibilities (Table 9-3). In the medical home model, NPs are eligible in some states to provide care, but may not be always designated as the "primary care provider."[10]

MCO Provider Enrollment

As with the indemnity insurer plan, separate inquiry to each MCO is required. Contact should be made through the provider relations department. Many MCOs may want the provider to be credentialed through Council for Affordable Quality Healthcare (CAQH). More details on CAQH are provided in the next section. The advantage of a CAQH application is that it eliminates multiple individual credentialing applications. In some states HMOs cannot discriminate against a provider based on their license. HMOs can accept or reject any provider.

When selecting which MCO to apply to, consideration is given to the MCOs who are utilized in your community or geographic area. You will also want to give consideration to their reimbursement practices both in amounts and how timely are they in their payments. You may need to negotiate a contract with the MCO. If there is an instance where contract negotiation is required, the use of an attorney who specializes in performing this service for NPs would be a recommendation. If you belong to a group practice, a member of the group will most likely be responsible for negotiating the terms of the MCO contract for the group.[10]

COUNCIL FOR AFFORDABLE QUALITY HEALTHCARE UNIVERSAL PROVIDER DATASOURCE

In 2012 the CAQH Universal Provider Datasource was created to simplify the provider credentialing process. The council is a free service to providers. The application is followed by an online attestation process (every 120 days). This application allows, with the completion of one form, credentialing for most managed care programs.[2] Once again, an updated CV is valuable to have on hand for the individual who is completing this application. Availability of license and certification numbers will also be required. Unfortunately, not all managed care programs allow NPs to be credentialed as providers. You should work with your state advanced practice organizations and the American Association of Nurse Practitioners to continue to lobby for NPs to be credentialed as individual and primary care providers. The website for CAQH is http://www.caqh.org/ (Table 9-4).[12]

AFFORDABLE CARE ACT—OBAMACARE

The Patient Protection and Affordable Care Act (PPACA), or as most of us know it by the Affordable Care Act (ACA) or its nickname Obamacare, was created in 2010 to improve access to care, expand coverage, control healthcare costs, and improve healthcare quality and care coordination.[13] In March 2011 provisions from the ACA were implemented requiring new provider screening and enrollment requirements for the Health Care Authority (HCA).

Affordable Care Act Provider Enrollment

There is no enrollment fee for individual physicians and individual non-physician providers and all providers enrolled under Medicare

TABLE 9-4

Information Required for CAQH Application
Educational chronology: entry and completion dates and address of academic setting
References: three professional
Employment chronology: beginning and termination dates and addresses
Hospital address and phone number, practice details: address, phone number, tax identification number, and National Provider Identifier number
Copies of educational diplomas, malpractice face sheet, basic or advanced life support cards
Malpractice information: name, address, and phone number. If claims—additional information will be required
Worker's compensation number
NP license number/Drug Enforcement Agency number, certificate to prescribe W-9
Billing contact information: address and phone number

or enrolled under another state's Medicaid. Specific details regarding enrollment requirements are available on the website at https://www.hca.wa.gov and https://www.ctdssmap.com.[14,15]

Filing claims for services provided in the ACA requires completion of the patient request for medical payment form (CMS-1490S). Specific instructions are provided based on the claim you are filing (i.e., Part B services, DME).[16]

SUMMARY

As NPs we are thankful for the passage of the Balanced Budget Act in 1997[6] which allowed NPs to have provider numbers and bill for services rendered. Receiving reimbursement for your services provided is a significant part of your revenue generation as an NP. Reimbursement for your services requires an initial application for an NPI number. After receiving your NPI number, you will be able to complete Medicare and Medicaid applications, indemnity insurers, MCOs, as well as a CAQH application. All of these applications are available online. The CAQH application requires an attestation every 120 days. The majority of insurance panels will allow you to apply right after you receive your license. There are a few that want a provider to have 2 or even 3 years of experience before being eligible to apply. This varies from state to state due to different regulations. The ability to be designated as a primary care provider also varies from plan to plan and state to state.

Careful attention to detail will minimize delays in obtaining these numbers that are significant for billing. Keeping a record of these insurance application numbers is as important as retaining your license numbers. These applications are usually completed by a practice manager or your billing service. They may be completed by individual providers as well. Being familiar with the different reimbursement sources is extremely beneficial at any time, and particularly if you are employed in a practice that has not had an NP provider previously.

References

1. National Plan and Provider Enumeration System. https://nppes.cms.hhs.gov/NPPES/Welcome.com. Accessed September 20, 2020.

2. Medicare Update. AANP Practice/Profession. https://www.aanp.org Accessed September 20, 2020.

3. Dillon D. & Hoyson P. (2014). Beginning Employment: A Guide for the New Nurse Practitioner. *The Journal for Nurse Practitioners*, 55–59.

4. usa.gov. https://www.usa.gov. Accessed September 20, 2020.

5. Centers for Medicare and Medicaid Services. https://www.cms.gov Accessed September 20, 2020.

6. H.R.2015—Balanced Budget Act of 1997—105th Congress. https://www.congress.gov/bill/105th-congress/house-105th-Congress-bill-2015 Accessed September 20, 2020.

7. Medicare Glossary. https://www.medicareresource.org. Accessed September 20, 2020.

8. Provider Enrollment, Chain, and Ownership System. https://pecos.cms.hhs.gov/pecos/login.com. Accessed September 20, 2020.

9. Medicaid. https://www.medicaid.gov. Accessed October 5, 2018.

10. Buppert, C. (2018). Reimbursement for Nurse Practitioner Services. In C. Buppert, editor. *Nurse Practitioner's Business Practice and Legal Guide* (p. 314). Burlington, MA: Jones & Bartlett Learning.

11. Indemnity Insurance Plans. https://www.ehealthinsurance.com. Accessed September 20, 2020.

12. Council for Affordable Quality Healthcare. http://www.caqh.org. Accessed September 20, 2020.

13. The Affordable Care Act. https://www.hhs.gov/opa/affordable-care-act. Accessed September 20, 2020.

14. The Affordable Care Act Provider Screening and Enrollment. http://www.hca.wa.gov. Accessed September 20, 2020.

15. Affordable Care Act (ACA) Provider Enrollment Requirements. https://www.ctdssmap.com. Accessed September 20, 2020.

16. Medicare.gov. How Do I File a Claim? https://www.medicare.gov. Accessed September 20, 2020.

10 Credentialing and Privileging

The next step in your employment process may require you to apply for healthcare system credentialing and privileging. This process is also part of the employment on-boarding for all hospital-based practitioners. The US Department of Health and Human Services definition for credentialing is "the process of assessing and confirming the qualifications of a licensed or certified health care provider."[1] The Joint Commission defines credentialing as "the process of obtaining, verifying, and assessing the qualifications of a practitioner to provide care or services in or for a health care organization."[2]

Credentialing is the first step to vet a provider for hospital practice. Credentialing for privileges is essential to ensure those providing services are qualified to do so. Over time, this process has become complicated due to the expansion of providers' scopes of practice, the requirements of third-party payers (e.g., the US government and private health insurance plans), and organizational standards of various accrediting bodies such as the Joint Commission.

Credentialing is a partner to privileging. Privileging is the process of authorizing a licensed or certified healthcare practitioner's specific scope of patient care services or scope of practice. Privileging is often performed in conjunction with an evaluation of an individual's clinical qualifications and/or performance.[3]

Hospital credentialing is required if your role requires you to see patients in the hospital setting or affiliated practices as part of your employment contract. Some of the managed care plans require their primary care providers to have hospital admitting privileges. In this instance you will be required to apply for privileges. This process is similar for all medical providers and is a requirement of the Joint Commission.[4]

Federal law requires that all hospitalized patients covered by Medicare must be under the care of a physician as a licensed doctor of medicine, osteopathy, dental surgery or dental medicine, podiatric medicine, chiropractic, or optometry.[5]

After a 1994 amendment was made to the Social Security Act to change federal Medicare law, clinical psychologists were added to the list of providers who may care for hospitalized patients.[5] An additional federal regulation allows physicians to "delegate tasks to other qualified healthcare personnel to the extent recognized under state law or a state's regulatory mechanism." It's this delegation regulation that NPs who deliver care to hospitalized patients fall under. While an NP may have admitting privileges, there must be a physician's name on the patient's record as "attending," in order to be compliant with this federal law.[6]

There are different levels of privileges that hospitals may assign to providers. Associate or affiliate staff privileges are often those granted to NPs. Associate/affiliate staff privileges are not full privileges. There are various limitations that can be imposed on providers with associate/affiliate staff privileges. Medical staff bylaws can also limit scope of practice for NP providers even if the privilege requested is within the NP's scope of practice and training. Full privileges are assigned to NPs and physician providers who have admitting privileges. Hospitals have medical staff bylaws and policies that define the various privileging levels.

THE PROCESS

The credentialing or on-boarding process itself is institution-dependent and may take from 90 days to 6 months to complete. Part of the process is initiated when you agree to accept the position applied for, have successfully passed your specific NP certification exam, and have received notification that you are licensed to practice in the state.

The process starts with a credentialing packet, or the delineation of clinical privileges packet, that is usually obtained from the medical staff office. Delineation of privileges is required by the Joint Commission. Do not be overwhelmed by the size of

TABLE 10-1

Hospital Credentialing
Background check—there may be a fee associated with this process
Continuing education hour log
Employment background—if there are gaps, be able to explain
Fingerprinting
National Practitioners Database inquiry
Nurse practitioner certification number
Practice information—address, phone number, fax number, contact person
Professional references—usually three
Collaborative practice agreement (if required by your practicing state)
State RN license number

this document. Hopefully this document will be in an electronic versus paper format. Medical administration staff are usually willing to assist you in the document completion. Completing this packet accurately and in its entirety is one key to expedite the process. There may be a fee required for submission of the completed packet. The cost of the credentialing packet submission may be the individual provider's or the group or practice may bear the cost. There is usually a fee associated with the application renewal process as well. This renewal fee may be annual or biannual. Table 10-1 identifies some of the items that may be required for the hospital credentialing process.

The preapplication process addresses the following:

- Disciplinary actions by licensing boards, payers, or professional organizations
- Unrestricted licensure
- Criminal history

- Board certification
- Clinical specialty
- Health status

Disciplinary Actions

State Boards of Nursing (State BON) where you have practiced will be contacted or their websites reviewed for any record of disciplinary actions or licensure restrictions. State BON are responsible for issuing and revoking licenses. State BON may also impose restrictions to practice on nursing licenses. Some of the common complaints to state BON that result in disciplinary action include breech in scope of practice, drug diversion or problematic alcohol use, ethical and moral issues or boundary violations, and criminal activity including felonies.[7]

Criminal Background Check

A criminal background check is performed as part of the credentialing process. The background check(s) may be required by both the Bureau of Criminal Investigation (BCI) and the Federal Bureau of Investigation (FBI). Both require fingerprinting. There may be an additional fee associated with the criminal background check. You will also have to address questions on the application related to this topic as well. Minor traffic violations are listed on the criminal background check. These violations are usually not addressed by the credentialing committee.

The National Practitioners Database (NPDB)

The NPDB inquiry serves as a repository of information about healthcare providers in the United States.[8] The program was developed in 1987 out of the Medicare and Medicaid Patient and Program Protection Act. The program was designed to protect program beneficiaries from unfit healthcare practitioners. Data that is reported to the database includes adverse licensure, hospital privilege, and professional society actions against physicians and dentists related to quality of care. In addition, the NPDB tracks malpractice payments/awards made for all healthcare practitioners.[8] State Boards of Nursing are required to report any adverse actions related to licensing or certification authority including revocation or suspension of a license reprimand, censure, or probation. The requirement is a reporting within 30 days of the action. Healthcare providers can perform a self-query to the database. As a new NP, in most instances, you will not have any reports in the database. Access to the NPDB is not available to the general public. Data stored in the NPDB is there permanently. Providers may submit addendums to their cases. A query to the NPDB is made on initial credentialing and on renewal applications.

Board Certification

Hospitals or agencies that credential NPs must also validate their board certification. This information can be obtained from the state Board of Nursing as well as the national certification body.

Health Status

Each facility will have its own way of asking for this information. Frequently it's a question on the credentialing application. The question is worded to the effect that do you have any existing health problems that could affect your ability to perform the requested privileges (i.e. substance abuse, alcohol use).

Curriculum Vitae (CV)

Information required to complete the credentialing packet often includes something similar to your CV. Additional documentation will be your license numbers with expiration dates as well as your NPI number. Having your updated CV in hand when completing the application will save you time. Make note of any gaps in your employment history. These are often "red flags" to the credentialing committee, the group of individuals assigned to review your privilege requests. Be prepared to explain the employment gaps as needed. Some acceptable reasons are looking for new employment, relocation, child or family care, or returning for continuing education.

Professional References

Professional references are required on the credentialing application. The reference letters are statements of your current competence as a provider. New graduate NPs will frequently request one of their professional references from a faculty member familiar with their educational and clinical experience. Other references may be obtained from clinical preceptors and colleagues who have worked with you. Before listing a name as a reference, be sure the individual has agreed to be a reference for you. Authorization to use someone as a reference before listing them on the application, as well as letting them know you are applying for a position, can and should be performed in advance. It's helpful to the individual completing the reference if you provide them some information on the position to which you are applying as well as some background information on yourself. This might expedite the return process on the letters of reference.

Other Necessary Documents

You will be required to furnish an updated continuing education log, collaborative practice agreement (if required by your state), as well as your RN and NP license numbers. Some facilities have a standard collaborative practice agreement that you can modify specific to your scope of practice. The collaborative practice agreement delineates how the NP and physician will work together in the clinical practice and the activities that can be performed autonomously as well as those which must be performed with physician collaboration. Be sure to inquire if the institution has their own collaborative practice agreement as this document will be the preferred agreement.

If you are requesting to perform procedures, you will need to furnish a procedure log to complete your delineation of privileges form. This log lists each procedure as well as how many times the procedure was performed by you. This list should outline if you performed the procedure in a simulation/lab setting, with a mentor/proctor, or performed independently. For new practitioners a copy of your Typhon log or other documentation from your NP program will be helpful. You may also be required to furnish educational proof that you have been trained to perform this procedure. A copy of your academic syllabus with the specific procedural content addressed is helpful to have to validate this education/training.

Primary source documentation, or credentials, such as copies of your graduation diploma(s), board certification, and any other RN certifications will also be requested. It's a good idea to make several copies of these documents before you have them framed and mounted for display. Insurance companies may also require copies of these documents for the insurance credentialing process.

Delays in the Process

Multiple items can delay the credentialing process. Some common reasons for application delays are incomplete applications, delays in receiving licensure notification from the board of nursing, and unreturned references. To minimize these delays (1) take time and effort to submit a complete and accurate credentialing application, (2) periodically check the board of nursing website for status updates and requests, and (3) contact individuals you are using for references in advance of submitting their names and provide follow-up phone calls as necessary.

OPPE and FPPE

Institutions will still require proctoring or supervision of specific procedures for a predetermined time interval as well. This is often referred to as a focused professional practice evaluation

(FPPE).[9] The FPPE and OPPE (ongoing professional practice evaluation) are components of a standard developed by the Joint Commission that a process be in place to evaluate clinical performance of the provider.[4] FPPE reviews are required on all new providers within 6 months of the granting of privileges, a significant patient event involving the provider, a critical patient complaint, or the request of a practice site based on ongoing practice concerns can also trigger an FPPE.[10] OPPE evaluation intervals are to be more frequent than annual. The frequency is determined by each individual facility. The Joint Commission requires that they are continuous, ongoing evaluations. The OPPE requires submission that the procedure was performed the minimal required times and the incidence of complications including morbidity. Requirements for minimal number of procedures required depend on the specific procedure as well as the institutional or recommended societal guidelines.

Insurance Credentialing

Depending on the practice arrangement, part of the hospital credentialing may include credentialing for various insurance providers. Having documents such as your CV and license number readily available and organized will save you significant time in this process. Details on the insurance credentialing process are included in Chapter 9.

Credentialing Committees

Once all of the information is received and the credentialing packet is complete, the information is forwarded to an internal credentialing committee. Frequently there is a credentialing committee specific for allied health professionals and a separate one for physician credentialing. The intradisciplinary committee is usually composed of several advanced practice nurses as well as physician members. The credentialing committee reviews the completed application as well as the request to perform any procedures. One function of the committee is to assure that the individual who is applying for privileges is requesting privileges that are within their scope of practice and educational training.

The next step in the credentialing process, after receiving approval from an Allied Health or similar committee, is to present the candidate's application to the hospital's Medical Executive Committee. You will receive a written notification from these committees regarding your credential status. You may also be scheduled to meet with the medical director at the completion of this process.

Both the Allied Health Committee and Medical Executive Committee have meetings that may be monthly, bimonthly, or quarterly. This is another factor that may impact on your actual start date as an NP. In most practice settings you cannot function as an NP in the hospital setting until this process is complete. Some facilities may grant "temporary or interim privileges."

Incidentals

An additional part of hospital credentialing is often referred to as the on-boarding process. During this process you will be provided with your identification badge, keys, and office. A plaque for your office door or your name on an existing nameplate is also appropriate. Parking passes or designated parking areas will be reviewed. If you have a position that requires an on-call schedule, inquire as to if there is specific parking available if you need to return to the practice setting after normal business hours.

Other things that may occur during this on-boarding process are receipt of a cellphone/pager, office phone number and fax, and email address. Some employers provide specific lab coats or scrubs. A review of the current dress code policy is also performed at this time. There should be a mechanism in place to introduce you to your new hospital community. Some facilities choose a newsletter or a specific department meeting. There may be posting of your picture on a specific website for NPs and physician providers.

Orientation or Fellowship

You will want to get details on the type and length of orientation that will be provided, as well as who is going to be your practice mentor. Will there be a specific NP or physician who will work with you and for what defined time frame? Having a positive relationship and communication with your mentor is one of the keys to a successful transition to your new NP role. A structured orientation or NP fellowship has also been shown to increase NP satisfaction and job retention. Training on the facilities' electronic health record is also part of an orientation. You may have been familiar with the electronic heath record as an RN, but the NP/provider record of the record is significantly different and requires a separate orientation.[11]

SUMMARY

An additional employment step for NPs who will be practicing in a healthcare system/hospital hospital setting is the credentialing and privileging process. Credentialing and privileging are considered part of the on-boarding process. This process can conjure up memories of your licensure application process. Although the process can be intimidating, having your documents organized and completed the first time the application is made will facilitate the granting of your privileging request. Utilizing the resources in the medical staff office can also lessen the frustration that can be associated with this process. When you receive written notification from the medical staff that your privileges have been approved, the credentialing process is completed. Once your on-boarding is complete, you will be officially allowed to start your practice of seeing patients. The recredentialing process is usually good for a 2-year time frame. It may be performed more frequently if the NP changes practice settings or requests additional procedures.

In today's world everyone wants to be assured that their provider is competent and appropriately trained. The hospital credentialing and privileging process may be one of many that you will be required to complete. It's a good idea to have readily available on a paper or electronic file recent copies of your CV, diploma, board certification certificate, licenses (i.e., RN, DEA), procedural logs, and letters of reference. Having these essential materials close at hand will help expedite your next credentialing process.

References

1. Health Resources and Services Administration. (2001, 2006). Credentialing and privileging of health center practitioners. Policy Information Notice 2001-6. https://bphc.hrsa.gov/policiesregulations/policies/pin200116.html. Accessed September 20, 2020.

2. Ambulatory Care Program: The Who, What, When, and Where's of Credentialing and Privileging. https://www.jointcommission.org. Accessed September 20, 2020.

3. Credentialing and Privileging. Medical Protective Clinical Risk Management Department. http://www.medpro.com/. Accessed September 20, 2020.

4. The Joint Accreditation Commission of Hospital Organizations. https://www.jointcommission.org. Accessed September 20, 2020.

5. Centers for Medicare and Medicaid Services, Department of Health and Human Services (2012). Medicare and Medicaid Programs: Reform of Hospital and Critical Access Hospital Conditions of Participation. *Federal Register,* 77 (95), 29034–29076.

6. Buppert, C. (2018). What Does It Mean to Have Hospital Privileges? In C. Buppert, editor, *Nurse Practitioner's Business Practice and Legal Guide* (pp. 267–268). Burlington, MA: Jones & Bartlett Learning.

7. Hudspeth, R. (2009). Understanding Discipline of Nurse Practitioners by Boards of Nursing. *The Journal for Nurse Practitioners,* 5 (5) 365–371.

8. National Practitioners Database. https://www.npdb.hrsa.gov. Accessed September 20, 2020.

9. High Reliability Healthcare. OPPE and FPPE: Tools to Help Make Privileging Decisions. https://www.jointcommission.org. 8/21/2013. Accessed September 20, 2020.

10. Joint Commission. (2011). *Standards BoosterPak for Focused Professional Practice Evaluation/Ongoing Professional Practice Evaluation.* Oakbrook Terrace, IL: The Joint Commission. http://2011.july.qualityandsafetynetwork.com. Accessed September 20, 2020.

11. Dillon, D., Dolansky, M., Casey, K., & Kelley, C. (2017). Factors Related to Successful Transition to Practice for Acute Care Nurse Practitioners. *AACN Advanced Critical Care,* 27 (2), 173–182.

11 Billing and Coding

INTRODUCTION

The billing and coding guidelines are jointly produced by the American Medical Association (AMA), the Department of Health and Human Services, and Centers for Medicare and Medicaid Services (CMS). NPs are encouraged to check the website periodically for updates and revisions at http://www.cms.gov. The revisions reproduced in this chapter were approved by the AMA and CMS in 2019.

You have been seeing patients throughout your entire NP program. Depending on the practice setting you were in you may have had a lot of exposure to billing and coding or a very limited and confusing exposure. If your NP program utilized a software program such as Typhon[1] you had exposure to some of the common Current Procedural Terminology (CPT) used in your specialty area. This information will continue to be helpful to you as you begin practice.

In the practice setting, some NPs continue to have limited exposure to billing and coding and have no idea how much revenue they might generate for their practice. One does not have to become a coder to understand the coding process and billing. Some new employee orientation programs will have a segment that includes some general coding information. There may also be follow-up sessions scheduled as you become familiar with your practice. You should also have access to resources in your practice.

There are currently five major categories of third-party payers. Each payer has its own provider application process, reimbursement policies, and fee schedules. Not all payers allow nonphysician providers to be credentialed or to be credentialed as primary care providers. Some payers have a fixed reimbursement for NPs, for example, 80%, regardless of physician presence in the office or physician consultation. The major third-party payers are Medicare, Medicaid, managed care organizations (MCOs), indemnity insurers, and direct contracts for health services by businesses. Depending on your NP population focus, you may interact with all or some of these payers.

There are many guidelines for billing and it is best to refer to the CMS[2] and other individual private payers for specific details. Some examples of billing guidelines refer to the first time a patient is seen to establish care. This visit must be billed under the NPs individual NPI number and those services are reimbursed at the 85% rate. This same guideline applies to established patients who present with a new medical problem—NPs individual NPI number and an 85% reimbursement rate. Other office setting patient visits may be billed under the "incident to" guideline as long as the physician in on site and the reimbursement is at 100%.[2] Billing guidelines also vary depending on site where service was performed (i.e., hospitals, skilled facilities, and hospice care).

In most practices the billing is performed by either an individual who may be an employee or a contracted service. Billing and coding are two separate functions. The coder deciphers the documentation of a patient interaction with the medical provider and determines the appropriate CPT® code and diagnosis to reflect the appropriate service provided. In the hospital setting coders often interact with providers to determine the most appropriate CPT® code to be utilized. The biller takes the assigned CPT® code and any other necessary information and enters them into a software program, submitting the claim to the insurance payer. The biller follows up on payment of the claim as necessary. The biller may also request additional information from you if this is requested by the insurance payer. Coders and billers can be a great resource for the NP. This is a complicated and ever-changing area.

CMS-1500/HCFA-1500

How do I bill or submit a claim? The standard document used for billing is the professional paper claim form known as the CMS-1500[2] or the HCFA-1500 which can be purchased from the AMA.[3] Specific information required on this form includes the date when the service was provided, ICD codes, CPT codes, patient identifying information, and provider identifying information. A bill submitted without the appropriate or incomplete information will be rejected. Although CMS-1500 is referred to as a professional paper claim the majority of claim submission is performed electronically with special software. You may daily submit the paper version which in turn the biller submits electronically.

IMPORTANCE OF BILLING AND CODING

Billing and coding are important from a variety of perspectives. Your reimbursement is a valuable contribution to your practice. "According to Medicare, only about 45% of all E/M (Evaluation and Management) claims are correct."[4] You want to be sure you code properly so that you receive the appropriate revenue that will be billed for the service you provided. Your documentation should have details to support the care provided or the procedure performed. You want to make sure you code appropriately based on your documentation. Similar to your documentation as an RN, the philosophy of "if it's not documented, it wasn't performed" holds true. Improper coding is considered fraud and can result in fines, paying monies back (or both), loss of licensure, and/or imprisonment. Proper coding starts with good documentation. Fraudulent billing can be in the form of both under and overbilling practices. Be sure to bill for what service(s) you provided. CMS notes that a joint effort between the healthcare provider and the coder is essential to achieve complete and accurate documentation, code assignment, and reporting of diagnoses and procedures.

CURRENT PROCEDURAL TERMINOLOGY (CPT®)

In order to submit a charge for the NP's services a basic understanding of the coding language is important. Current procedural terminology, or CPT® coding for short, is the common language used by medical providers and insurance carriers to identify and bill for medical services and procedures. CPT® is a registered

TABLE 11-1

Category 1—CPT Coding
Evaluation and management
Anesthesiology
Surgery
Radiology
Pathology and laboratory
Medicine

trademark of the AMA.[3] The AMA and CMS develop the codes, descriptions, and guidelines that describe the procedures and services performed by physicians and other healthcare providers. These codes are then adopted by Medicare and third-party payers. Each provider and Medicare have a corresponding fee attached to each CPT® code. CPT® codes are used in combination with the ICD-10 CM numerical diagnostic coding.

There are three types of CPT® codes currently used. They are known as Category 1, Category 2, and Category 3. Most of your exposure will be with the Category 1 codes. Category 1 codes (Table 11-1) are those procedures and contemporary medical practices that are commonly performed. They are five-digit numeric codes that identify the service or the procedure that is Food and Drug Administration (FDA) approved, and performed by providers nationwide and is proven and documented.

Category 2 is a CPT® medical code set that consists of supplementary tracking codes that are used for performance measures and are intended to help collect information about the quality of care delivered. The use of this medical code set is considered optional. Category 2 CPT® codes are not a substitute for a Category 1 code.

The Category 3 CPT® codes are considered temporary codes. They are not widely used services and procedures. They are frequently used for services and procedures that are new and emerging technologies and have not yet received FDA approval.

The service or procedure may also not have any proven clinical efficacy at this point in time. The Category 3 CPT® codes are what are used for research. The purpose of the Category 3 CPT® codes is to help researchers track emerging technologies and services.[5]

EVALUATION AND MANAGEMENT (E/M)

E/M codes represent the NPs cognitive services, office/clinic visits, consultations, preventative medical examination, and critical care services.[6] These are the codes used for reimbursement when you perform a history, physical examination, arrive at a diagnosis and then recommend a treatment plan. To receive payment for service you provided the service must be within the scope of practice for the relevant type of provider in the state in which they are furnished.[7] E/M services are billed depending on where the service is provided. Office or other outpatient settings, inpatient hospital, emergency department, and nursing facilities are examples of sites of service. The code sets to bill for E/M are organized into various categories and levels. As an example, the more complex the visit, the higher the level of code utilized. Selecting the appropriate code must reflect the service provided.

E/M consists of the following five components for established patients: history taking, performance of physical examination, medical decision making, counseling, and coordination of care The number of levels was reduced to 4 for office/outpatient E/M visits for new patients and definitions were revised in 2020. There is a 2020 Medicare Physician Fee Schedule Final Rule that is requesting a revised requirement for this billing and CMS will no longer collapse level 2-4 E/M visits into one blended payment. The history consists of the chief complaint, the history of the present illness, the review of systems, and the patient's past medical history, family history, and social history. The CPT code changes allow providers to choose the E/M visit level based on either medical decision making or time.

CHIEF COMPLAINT

The chief complaint is always a required part of the provider's documentation regardless of the type or level of encounter. It is best stated in the patient's own words when possible. It is the patient's description of what is going on. In length, the chief complaint may range from a few words to one or two short sentences. For example, "after my fall my left leg is hurting".

HISTORY OF THE PRESENT ILLNESS (HPI)

HPI is frequently described using nomograms such as OLDCARTS (**O**nset, **l**ocation, **d**uration, **c**haracteristics, **a**ggravating or **r**elieving factors, **t**reatments, and **s**everity) or PQRST (**P**rovocative or **P**alliative, **Q**uality or **Q**uantity, **R**egion or **R**adiation, **S**everity, and **T**iming).

HPIs can either be a **brief HPI** using only three elements (e.g., onset, duration, and characteristics) or an **extended/comprehensive HPI** which uses at least four (e.g., onset, location, duration, characteristics, severity) of the above elements.

There are four types of histories. To qualify for a specific type of history, all four elements indicated in Table 11-2 must be met.[7]

TABLE 11-2

Benefits of FPA

Type of history	Chief complaint	HPI	ROS	PFSH
Problem focused	Required	Brief	N/A	N/A
Expanded problem focused	Required	Brief	Problem pertinent	N/A
Detailed	Required	Extended	Extended	Pertinent
Comprehensive	Required	Extended	Complete	Complete

Example: HPI from the chief complaint identified above "after my fall my left leg is hurting."

Onset: Fall occurred 2 days prior to office visit

Location: Left lower extremity pain

Duration: Pain occurred immediately with the fall

Characteristics: Describes the pain as aching and can pinpoint the area of pain

Aggravating: Pain is worse with standing and at night while trying to sleep

Relieving factors: Heat and Tylenol provide some relief

Timing: Pain is constant

Severity: On a scale of 1 to 10 patient identifies pain as an eight

REVIEW OF SYSTEMS (ROS)

The ROS is performed by a systematic interview of the body systems. Commonly recognized ROS are given in Table 11-3.

There are considered to be three types of ROS: problem pertinent ROS, extended ROS, and a complete ROS.

Problem Pertinent ROS

This includes only inquiries regarding the system involved in the chief complaint and HPI. Using the example of chest pain, one system, cardiovascular is reviewed.

Extended ROS

This includes information regarding the system involved in the HPI and a limited number of additional two to nine systems.

Complete ROS

This includes information regarding the system involved in the HPI as well as an additional 10 to 12 systems (Table 11-4).

TABLE 11-3

Common Systems for the Review of Systems

• Constitutional symptoms—weight loss, fever, fatigue
• Allergic/Immunologic
• Cardiovascular
• Endocrine
• Gastrointestinal
• Genitourinary
• HEENT—head, eyes, ears, nose, and throat
• Hematologic/Lymphatic
• Integumentary
• Musculoskeletal
• Neurological
• Psychiatric
• Pulmonary

TABLE 11-4

Examples of the Three Types of Review of Systems with the Chief Complaint of "I'm Having Chest Pain"

Problem pertinent ROS: Review of cardiovascular system

Extended ROS: Review of cardiovascular system and gastrointestinal systems

Complete ROS: Review of constitutional complaints, allergic cardiovascular, endocrine gastrointestinal, hematologic, musculoskeletal, neurologic, and respiratory

PAST MEDICAL HISTORY, FAMILY HISTORY, AND SOCIAL HISTORY (PFSH)

The past medical history refers to the patient's prior experiences with illness, injuries, and treatments. Frequently you will see the surgical history listed separately in this section. Dates associated with the past medical history should also be listed when possible. Significant minor surgeries are traditionally only listed if occurred in the prior 5 years (i.e., tonsillectomy at age 4—patient is now 60). Major surgical procedures (e.g., open heart surgery) are always listed regardless of the date the procedure was performed.

The family history is where significant family medical problems are identified. These may be hereditary diseases. It is also significant to identify what member of the family experienced the illness and at what age was the diagnosis made. A mother with a history of breast cancer at age 40 provides more information than just listing breast cancer as a family medical problem. The family history should include history that is significant in parents, grandparents, siblings, aunts, and uncles.

The social history can include information related to marital status, living conditions, travel, and habits (e.g., substance abuse, tobacco/vaping and alcohol use/abuse). The social history is age appropriate. Questions in this area can be sensitive and in order to obtain the information you are desiring, need to be asked with skill and empathy.

The information obtained in the PFSH may be obtained by the patient completing a questionnaire type medical document or by a medical assistant or other support staff collecting the data. It must be documented that the NP reviewed the data and updated as indicated. It is not necessary for the NP to collect the data themselves. You should be familiar with what data is required in the PFSH portion of the history taking, and be able to supplement this data as needed.

For coding purposes at least one item from two of the three areas (past medical history, family history, or social history) must be documented to be considered a **pertinent PFSH**. A **complete PFSH** is a review of two or all three of the areas.

THE PHYSICAL EXAMINATION

The physical examination may involve a single organ (Table 11-5) or multiple organ systems (Table 11-6). These examinations may be problem focused, expanded problem focused, detailed, or comprehensive.

The Evaluation and Management Services Guide[7] identifies several important points to keep in mind when documenting general multisystem and single organ system examinations.

- Document specific abnormal and relevant negative findings of the examination of the affected or symptomatic body area(s) or organ system(s). A notation of "abnormal" without elaboration is not sufficient.
- Describe abnormal or unexpected findings of the examination of any asymptomatic body area(s) or organ system(s).
- It is sufficient to provide a brief statement or notation indicating "negative" or "normal" to document normal findings related to unaffected area(s) or asymptomatic organ system(s).

MEDICAL DECISION MAKING

Medical decision making is the next step in the coding process. Medical decisions are based on their complexity to be minimum, low, moderate, or high complexity. The highest level of risk in any of the categories determines the overall risk (Table11-7).

Medical decision making refers to the complexity of establishing a diagnosis and/or selecting a management option, which is determined by considering the following factors:

- The number of possible diagnoses and/or the number of management options that must be considered.

TABLE 11-5

Single-Organ System Examination

Type of examination	Description
Problem focused	Include performance and documentation of one to five elements identified by a bullet in one or more organ system(s) or body area(s)
Expanded problem focused	Include performance and documentation of at least six elements identified by a bullet in one or more organ system(s) or body area(s)
Detailed	Examinations other than the eye and psychiatric examinations should include performance and documentation of at least 12 elements identified by a bullet, whether in a box with a shaded or unshaded border. Eye and psychiatric examinations include the performance and documentation of at least nine elements identified by a bullet, whether in a box with a shaded or unshaded border
Comprehensive	Include performance of all elements identified by a bullet, whether in a shaded or unshaded box. Documentation of every element in each box with a shaded border and at least one element in a box with an unshaded border is expected

Both types of examinations may be performed by any physician, regardless of specialty. Here are some important points to keep in mind when documenting general multisystem and single-organ system examinations (in both the 1995 and the 1997 documentation guidelines): Document specific abnormal and relevant negative findings of the examination of the affected or symptomatic body area(s) or organ system(s). A notation of "abnormal" without elaboration is not sufficient. Describe abnormal or unexpected findings of the examination of any asymptomatic body area(s) or organ system(s). ™It is sufficient to provide a brief statement or notation indicating "negative" or "normal" to document normal findings related to unaffected area(s) or asymptomatic organ system(s).

Source: Reproduced from the CMS.

TABLE 11-6

General Multisystem Examination

Type of examination	Description
Problem focused	Include performance and documentation of one to five elements identified by a bullet in one or more organ system(s) or body area(s)
Expanded problem focused	Include performance and documentation of at least six elements identified by a bullet in one or more organ system(s) or body area(s)
Detailed	Include at least Include at least two elements identified by a bullet from each of six areas/systems OR at least twelve elements identified by a bullet in two or more areas/systems.
Comprehensive	Include at least nine organ systems or body areas. For each system/area selected, all elements of the examination identified by a bullet should be performed, unless specific directions limit the content of the examination. For each area/system documentation of at least two elements identified by bullet is expected *

*The 1997 documentation guidelines state that the medical record for a general multisystem examination should include findings about eight or more organ systems.
Source: Reproduced from reference 7.

- The amount and/or complexity of medical records, diagnostic tests, and/or other information that must be obtained, reviewed, and analyzed.
- The risk of significant complications, morbidity, and/or mortality as well as comorbidities associated with the patient's presenting problem(s), the diagnostic procedure(s), and/or the possible management options.

TABLE 11-7

Medical Decision Making

Type of decision making—level of risk	Presenting problem(s)	Diagnostic testing/procedure(s) ordered	Management option selected
Minimum complexity (minimal)	One self-limited problem (e.g., cold, insect bite, tinea corporis)	Laboratory tests EKG/EEG CXR Urinalysis Ultrasound/Echocardiogram KOH prep	Rest Gargles Elastic bandages Superficial dressings
Low complexity	Two or more self-limited problems or minor problem (e.g., hypertension, diabetes) One stable chronic illness Acute, uncomplicated illness or injury (e.g., cystitis, allergic rhinitis, simple sprain)	2 Physiologic tests not under stress (e.g., pulmonary function tests) Noncardiovascular imaging studies with contrast (e.g., barium enema) Superficial needle biopsies Clinical laboratory tests requiring arterial puncture Skin biopsies	Minor surgery with no identified risk factors Over-the-counter-drugs Physical therapy Occupational therapy IV fluids without additives

Moderate complexity	3	One or more chronic illnesses with mild exacerbation Two or more stable chronic illnesses Acute illness with systemic symptoms (e.g., pyelonephritis, pneumonitis, colitis) Acute complicated injury (e.g., head injury with brief loss of consciousness)	Physiologic tests under stress (e.g., cardiac stress test, fetal contraction stress test) Diagnostic endoscopies with no identified risk factors Deep needle or incisional biopsies CV imaging studies with contrast and no identified risk factors (e.g., arteriogram, cardiac catheterization) Obtain fluid from body cavity (e.g., lumbar puncture, thoracentesis, culdocentesis)	Minor surgery with identified risk factors Elective major surgery (open, percutaneous, or endoscopic) with no identified risk factors Prescription drug management Therapeutic nuclear medicine IV fluids with additives Closed treatment of fracture or dislocation without manipulation
High complexity	4	One or more chronic illnesses with severe exacerbation, progression, or side effects of treatment Abrupt change in neurological status (e.g., seizure, TIA, weakness, sensory loss)	Cardiovascular imaging studies with contrast with identified risk factors Cardiac electrophysiological tests Diagnostic endoscopies with identified risk factors Discography	Elective major surgery (open, percutaneous, or endoscopic) with identifiable risk factors Emergency major surgery (open, percutaneous, or endoscopic) Parenteral controlled substances Drug therapy requiring intensive monitoring for toxicity Decision not to resuscitate or de-escalate care because of poor prognosis

Source: Compiled from the CMS.[7,10]

As a general rule, decision making for a diagnosed problem is easier than decision making for an identified but undiagnosed problem. The number and type of diagnosed tests performed may be an indicator of the number of possible diagnoses. Problems that are improving or resolving are less complex than those problems that are worsening or failing to change as expected. Another indicator of the complexity of diagnostic or management problems is the need to seek advice from other healthcare professionals.[7]

There are some important points to keep in mind when documenting the number of diagnoses or management options. You should document:

- An assessment, clinical impression, or diagnosis for each encounter, which may be explicitly stated or implied in documented decisions for management plans and/or further evaluation.
- For a presenting problem with an established diagnosis, the record should reflect whether the problem is:
  - Improved, well controlled, resolving, or resolved
  - Inadequately controlled, worsening, or failing to change as expected
- For a presenting problem without an established diagnosis, the assessment or clinical impression may be stated in the form of differential diagnoses or as a "possible," "probable," or "rule out" diagnosis
- The initiation of, or changes in, treatment, which includes a wide range of management options such as patient instructions, nursing instructions, therapies, and medications.
- If referrals are made, consultations requested, or advice sought, to whom or where the referral or consultation is made or from whom advice is requested.

AMOUNT AND/OR COMPLEXITY OF DATA TO BE REVIEWED

The amount and/or complexity of data to be reviewed is based on the types of diagnostic testing ordered or reviewed. Indications of the amount and/or complexity of data being reviewed include:

- A decision to obtain and review old medical records and/or obtain history from sources other than the patient (increases the amount and complexity of data to be reviewed).

- Discussion of contradictory or unexpected test results with the physician who performed or interpreted the test (indicates the complexity of data to be reviewed).

- The physician who ordered a test personally reviews the image, tracing, or specimen to supplement information from the physician who prepared the test report or interpretation (indicates the complexity of data to be reviewed).

Here are some important points to keep in mind when documenting amount and/or complexity of data to be reviewed. You should document:

- The type of service, if a diagnostic service is ordered, planned, scheduled, or performed at the time of the E/M encounter.

- The review of laboratory, radiology, and/or other diagnostic tests. A simple notation such as "WBC elevated" or "Chest x-ray unremarkable" is acceptable. Alternatively, document the review by initialing and dating the report that contains the test results.

- A decision to obtain old records or additional history from the family, caretaker, or other source to supplement information obtained from the patient.

- Relevant findings from the review of old records and/or the receipt of additional history from the family, caretaker, or other source to supplement information obtained from the patient. You should document that there is no relevant information beyond that already obtained, as appropriate. A notation of "old records reviewed" or "additional history obtained from family" without elaboration is not sufficient.

- Discussion about results of laboratory, radiology, or other diagnostic tests with the physician who performed or interpreted the study.

- The direct visualization and independent interpretation of an image, tracing, or specimen previously or subsequently interpreted by another physician.

RISK OF SIGNIFICANT COMPLICATIONS, MORBIDITY, AND/OR MORTALITY

The risk of significant complications, morbidity, and/or mortality is based on the risks associated with these categories:

- Presenting problem(s)
- Diagnostic procedure(s)
- Possible management options

The assessment of risk of the presenting problem(s) is based on the risk related to the disease process anticipated between the present encounter and the next encounter.

The assessment of risk of selecting diagnostic procedures and management options is based on the risk during and immediately following any procedures or treatment. The highest level of risk in any one category determines the overall risk.

The level of risk of significant complications, morbidity, and/or mortality can be:

- Minimal
- Low
- Moderate
- High

TABLE 11-8

Elements for Each Level of Medical Decision Making

Type of decision making	Number of diagnoses or management options	Amount and/or complexity of data to be reviewed	Risk of complications, morbidity, and/or mortality
Straightforward	Minimal	Minimal or none	Minimal
Low complexity	Limited	Limited	Low
Moderate complexity	Multiple	Moderate	Moderate
High complexity	Extensive	Extensive	High

Here are some important points to keep in mind when documenting level of risk. You should document:

- Comorbidities/underlying diseases or other factors that increase the complexity of medical decision making by increasing the risk of complications, morbidity, and/or mortality.
- The type of procedure, if a surgical or invasive diagnostic procedure is ordered, planned, or scheduled at the time of the E/M encounter.
- The specific procedure, if a surgical or invasive diagnostic procedure is performed at the time of the E/M encounter.
- The referral for or decision to perform a surgical or invasive diagnostic procedure on an urgent basis. This point may be implied.

Table 11-8 can help determine whether the level of risk of significant complications, morbidity, and/or mortality is minimal, low, moderate, or high. Because determination of risk is complex and not readily quantifiable, the table includes common clinical examples rather than absolute measures of risk. Let's take this through the process with a patient example. Mr. J, a 55-year-old male, who presents to the office with the chief complaint "I sprained my left ankle." He acknowledges playing baseball with grandchildren last evening. He notes some bruising and swelling. He has been applying ice. You have examined him and determined this is a simple sprain. No further workup is needed unless the symptom does not improve.

The level of risk is **low** as this is considered a simple sprain (2 Points)

Diagnostic procedures ordered—none (0 Points)

Management option selected—elastic bandage or ace wrap (1 Point)

Given the above information his presenting problem point is a 2, zero points for diagnostic procedures ordered and zero points as no data was reviewed. This is a total of 2 points and the visit qualifies as low-risk patient encounter.

DOCUMENTATION OF AN ENCOUNTER DOMINATED BY COUNSELING AND/OR COORDINATION OF CARE

When counseling and/or coordination of care dominates (more than 50%) the physician/patient and/or family encounter (face-to-face time in the office or other outpatient setting, floor/unit time in the hospital, or NF), time is considered the key or controlling factor to qualify for a particular level of E/M services. If the level of service is reported based on counseling and/or coordination of care, you should document the total length of time of the encounter and the record should describe the counseling and/or activities to coordinate care. The Level I and Level II CPT® books, available from the AMA, list average time guidelines for a variety of E/M services. These times include work done before, during, and after the encounter. The specific times expressed in the code descriptors are averages and, therefore, represent a range of times that may be higher or lower depending on actual clinical circumstances.

OTHER CONSIDERATIONS

Split/Shared Services

A split/shared service is an encounter where a physician and an NP each personally perform a portion of an E/M visit. Here are the rules for reporting split/shared E/M services between physicians and NPs:

- In the office or clinic setting:
  - For encounters with established patients who meet incident to requirements, use either practitioner's National Provider Identifier (NPI)
  - For encounters that do not meet incident to requirements, use the NPs NPI
- Hospital inpatient, outpatient, and ED setting encounters shared between a physician and an NP from the same group practice:
  - When the physician provides any face-to-face portion of the encounter, use either provider's NPI
  - When the physician does not provide a face-to-face encounter, use the NPP's NPI

Consultation Services

Effective for services furnished on or after January 1, 2010, Medicare no longer recognizes inpatient consultation codes (CPT codes 99251–99255) and office and other outpatient consultation codes (CPT codes 99241–99245) for Part B payment purposes. However, Medicare recognizes telehealth consultation codes (HCPCS G0406–G0408 and G0425–G0427) for payment. Physicians and NPs who furnish services that, prior to January 1, 2010, would have been reported as CPT consultation codes, should report the appropriate E/M visit code to bill for these services beginning January 1, 2010.[7]

Time Spent

One final variable is the time spent face-to-face with the patient. The NP may choose to bill based on time spent versus billing based on history, physical examination, and medical decision making. This is acceptable in certain instances where the face-to-face encounter is dominated by counseling and/or care coordination (50% or more).[11] When time spent is utilized as the method for coding, there are no specific documentation requirements. It is recommended, however, that the NP record this information in the medical record. There are predetermined times assigned to different levels of visits (e.g., new patient, existing patient, inpatient, outpatient). It is crucial that the time spent face-to-face with the patient be documented. An example of this type of documentation could be: A total of 30 minutes was spent in a face-to-face discussion with the patient regarding their hypertension management of which 50% of that time was spent on counseling and coordination of care. The patient was educated on lifestyle modifications including diet, exercise, and weight loss.

Medicare and CPT® differ when it comes to determining the time to report for encounters for which the provider spends more than half of the visit counseling or coordinating the care of the patient. CPT® allows the provider to round up when reporting the provider's time, whereas Medicare does not.[10]

An example of this in the *CPT® Manual* code descriptions, the typical time code for 99213 is 15 minutes and 10 minutes for Code 99212. For CMS, when the provider documents that he or she spend more than 50% of the 13-minute visit with the patient discussing the treatment options, the code should be reported as 99212, not 99213. For this same encounter, CPT® guidelines allow providers to round up and report CPT® code 99212.[11]

ICD-10 Coding

ICD-10 stands for International Disease Coding version 10.[12] ICD-10-PCS stands for Procedure Coding System and is composed of seven characters. Each character is an axis of classification that specifies information about the procedure performed. ICD-10 coding enables you to specifically classify diseases, functioning, and disability. CMS launched the new ICD-10 coding in October 2015. As compared to the previous ICD-9 coding, there are at least 1/3 more available codes. The codes allow the provider to be more specific. Two examples of more specific coding are as follows. In the visit example with the patient with a sprained ankle, the new ICD-10 code would allow for laterality—choosing right versus left in this example. When describing a patient with Type II diabetes mellitus now, rather than just, T2DM, you should add uncontrolled, with renal complications—if appropriate for your patient. With the move toward "pay for performance," this becoming more specific in your coding will improve the opportunity to be paid better if you are able to improve these metrics. When you code a visit be sure the ICD-10 code is consistent with the E/M code. You will create a "red flag" if you bill for a high-level visit and then use an ICD-10 code that is not consistent. If you choose to bill the high-level visit with an ICD-10 code that may draw attention, be sure your documentation supports the visit in the event of an insurance audit.

CMS CHANGES

CMS has been performing a listening campaign with providers and proposing in its annual changes to reduce the burden of excess documentation, thereby allowing clinicians to spend more time with their patients and focus on documenting the most important parts of a visit.[13] As you have probably observed with your preceptors, documentation is critical and time consuming. Often you will witness them performing the details of documentation after patient visits have been completed. The use of the electronic medical record for documentation has posed new challenges for providers with this documentation being performed while in the patient's presence. There is a skill to develop in performing this function so the patient does not feel they are not significant and to assure that you do not miss important details of the patient visit.

To reduce burden, CMS finalized modifications to their documentation policy so that physicians, physician assistants, and advanced practice registered nurses can review and verify (sign and date), rather than re-documenting, notes made in the medical record by other physicians, residents, medical, physician assistant and APRN students, nurses, or other members of the medical team.

Some of the changes made in 2020 were discussed under E/M services with the 5 levels of coding for established patients and the reduction to 4 levels for office/outpatient E/M visits for new patients with revised code definitions. The CPT code changes revised the times and medical decision-making processes for all of the codes, and requires performance of history and exam only as medically appropriate. The remaining CPT change allows for providers to choose the E/M visit level based on either medical decision making or time.

VALUE-BASED CARE—QUALITY PAYMENT PROGRAM (QPP)

Medicare's QPP is another determination that expects had changes in 2020. Medicare and commercial payers have moved toward a value-based payment system over the past several years. Value-based payment moves from the payment method based on volume of care, such as is seen in the traditional fee-for-service model. Instead of payment based on a higher volume of patients seen, the value-based payment model measures quality and cost to determine payment made to providers. The value-based payment method is a way to ensure high-quality care while attempting to control cost. Value-based care is an attempt to equalize payments between office and hospital-based providers. Value-based care arrangements may also permit providers to address social determinants of health, as well as disparities across the healthcare system.

CMS expanded the exclusion criteria for 2019 to include one of the following:

- **Threshold was added:** 1) furnishing less than or equal to $90,000 in Medicare Part B covered professional services; 2) furnishing covered professional services to 200 or fewer Medicare beneficiaries; 3) or furnishing 200 or fewer covered professional services.

- **Ability to opt into the merit-based incentive payment system (MIPS).** Clinicians and groups that meet or exceed at least one of these criteria will be excluded from MIPS unless they affirmatively opt in. In 2019 CMS finalized an opt-in policy that allows eligible clinicians to opt-in to MPIS if the eligible clinician or group meets or exceeds at least one, but not all, of the low-volume threshold criteria. Once a decision to opt-in is communicated to CMS, it cannot be reversed.

- **Changes to general performance category weights used to calculate MIPS scores.** Quality decreased to 45%. Promoting Interoperability is 25%. Improvement activities changed to 15%. Cost is 15% as well. Promoting interoperability (formerly called advancing care information) and improvement activities remain at 25% and 15% of the total score, respectively. MIPS eligible clinicians and groups must achieve at least 30 points to avoid a reimbursement penalty of 7 percent and at least 75 points to be eligible for a positive reimbursement adjustment. [14]

- **Removal of 34 quality measures deemed by CMS to be of low value.** [15]

- **Requiring the use of 2015 edition certified EHR technology in 2019.** This was originally proposed for 2018, but CMS backtracked to allow 2014 edition certification because EHR vendors were not ready.[14]

A major change proposed in the physician fee schedule was a restructure E/M codes. Previously, office-based providers code for five different levels of care, with different codes and reimbursement rates for new and established patients. The coding is based on the complexity of the visit. Under the recent change, E/M levels 2 to 5 were combined into one payment rate, with add-on codes included to address visits of greater complexity. The potential impact is that office-based providers who see more patients with less complex health issues (levels 1 to 3) could see reimbursement rates rise, while physicians who deal largely with levels 4 to 5 complexity could see reimbursement rates decrease.[15]

Other New changes are reimbursement for "technology-based services." These services are outside of the telemedicine services that are already reimbursed. These technology-based services include a brief, non-face-to-face check-in with a patient via phone, text messages, email, or video conferencing to evaluate whether the patient needs to be seen in the office. Previously, these services required a significant amount of time and were not reimbursable. In response to the COVID-19 pandemic, CMS moved swiftly to significantly expand payment for telehealth services and implement other flexibilities so that Medicare beneficiaries living in all areas of the country could get convenient and high-quality care from the comfort of their home while avoiding unnecessary exposure to the virus.

CARE MANAGEMENT SERVICES

In calendar year 2020 proposals are being finalized for transitional care management (TCM). These are services that are provided to beneficiaries after discharge from and inpatient stay or certain outpatient stays.

A Medicare specific code in being created for additional time spent beyond the initial 20 minutes allowed in the current coding for chronic care management services.

SUMMARY

Detailed documentation is the first step to accurate billing and coding. Understanding what is the required documentation for each patient encounter is significant. This is a continual learning process. Taking the time to document the care you have provided not only is evidence of best care practices but facilitates the review of your documentation by coders and insurance carriers. It is supported by the continued philosophy, "if it's not documented, it wasn't performed." Supporting your visit coding level with appropriate documentation will save you both time and money. It is also a good legal defense of the care you provided. Utilizing the resources of both billers and coders can help you develop your skills and expertise in this area.

Remember, you should be the only one coding your visit. No one should make changes to your coding sheet without your approval. Again, you are responsible for the billing done on your behalf, so have a clear understanding of what is being done by a coder or your billing company if changes are made. Continually staying abreast of changes in documentation and coding is an ongoing process in view of CMS annual fee schedule updates. One thing is always guaranteed that change is certain and constant.

References

1. Typhon Group LLC. http://www.typhongroup.com. Accessed September 19, 2020.

2. Centers for Medicare and Medicaid Services. https://www.cms.gov. Accessed September 19, 2020.

3. American Medical Association. http://www.ama-assn.org/. Accessed September 19, 2020.

4. Williams, L. http://www.coding-advisor.com, Accessed September 19, 2020.

5. Rouse, M. *Definition Current Procedural Terminology (CPT)*. Retrieved from SearchHealthIT. http://www.searchhealthit.techtarget.com. Accessed September 19, 2020.

6. Buppert, C. (2018). *Reimbursement for Nurse Practitioners in Nurse Practitioners Business and Legal Guide* (p. 320). 6th ed. Burlington, MA: Jones and Bartlett Learning.

7. *Evaluation and Management Services Guide (ICN 006764)*. (2020, January). Baltimore, MD: U.S. Centers for Medicare and Medicaid Services (CMS).

8. American Association of Nurse Practitioners. AANP.Centers for Medicare and Medicaide-aanp,org/advocacy/federal/federal-regulation. Accessed September 21, 2020.

9. Evaluation and Management (E/M) Services. cms.gov/newsroom/fact-sheets/finalized-policy-payment-and-quality-provisions-changes-medicare-physician-fee-schedule-calendar. Accessed September 22.2020

10. *Medicare Claims Processing Manual*. Chapter 12, Section 30.6.15.1. Baltimore, MD: U.S. Centers for Medicare and Medicaid Services (CMS). September 19, 2020. (Rev. 4431).

11. Bolarakis, S. (2009, December 16). CMS and AMA Documentations Guidelines for E/M Codes Don't Always Agree. *JustCoding News: Outpatient*.

12. ICD-10 codes. International Classification of Diseases. www.cdc.gov/nchs/icd/icd10cm.htm. Accessed September 19, 2020.

13. Proposed Changes to Evaluation and Management (E/M) Billing for Medicare Beneficiaries. American Association of Nurse Practitioners. https://www.aanp.org. Accessed September 19, 2020.

14. 2019 MIPS strategic scoring card. American Medical Associations. ama-assn.org/system/files/2019-05-2019-MIPS-scoring-guide.pdf. Accessed September 20, 2020.

15. 4 ways Doctor Reimbursement Could Change Next Year. Medical Economics Staff. https://www.medicaleconomics.com. Accessed September 19, 2020.

12 Full Practice Authority

Full Practice Authority (FPA) as defined by the American Association of Nurse Practitioners (AANP) is "the collection of state practice and licensure laws that allow for nurse practitioners to evaluate patients, diagnose, order and interpret diagnostic tests, initiate and manage treatments—including the ability to prescribe medications—under exclusive licensure authority of the state board of nursing."[1] AANP supports the modernization of state licensure laws. This licensure model, Full Practice Authority, is supported by decades of evidence and is recommended by the National Council of State Boards of Nursing (NCSBN), the National Academy of Medicine (formerly the IOM), and other leading health policy experts. The country continues to experience a restriction in scope of practice for nurse practitioners (NPs) which remains costly to the economy and presents a barrier to patient care. Currently states, plus the District of Columbia, and two US territories (Guam and the Marianas Islands). permit NPs to diagnose, treat, and prescribe medications without physician oversight—Full Practice Authority (Figure 12-1). In 2008, the Robert Wood Johnson Foundation (RWJF) partnered with the Institute of Medicine (IOM)* to establish an Initiative on *The Future of Nursing: Leading Change, Advancing Health.*

In 2010 the committee released its landmark report that recommended scope-of-practice (SOP) barriers should be removed to allow advanced practice registered nurses (APRNs) to practice to the full extent of their education and training.[2]

Assessments have been made on the IOM report, *The Future of Nursing.*[2] In 2011, the American Nurses Association (ANA) released a statement in which the organization and its members were actively pursuing change, such as the efforts of state nursing associations to make state-level changes to SOP laws.[3] In 2014, the Federal Trade Commission (FTC) released a paper stating, "physician supervision requirements may raise competition concerns because they effectively give one group

---

*The IOM is now known by its new name the National Academy of Medicine.

FIGURE 12-1 AANP 2021 Nurse Practitioner State Practice Environment

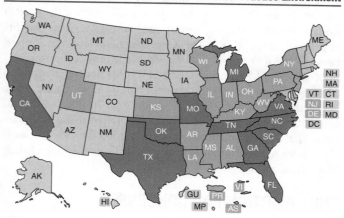

Full Practice: State practice and licensure laws permit all NPs to evaluate patients; diagnose, order and interpret diagnostic tests; and initiate and manage treatments, including prescribing medications and controlled substances, under the exclusive licensure authority of the state board of nursing. This is the model recommended by the National Academy of Medicine, formerly called the Institute of Medicine, and the National Council of State Boards of Nursing.

Reduced Practice: State practice and licensure laws reduce the ability of NPs to engage in at least one element of NP practice. State law requires a career-long regulated collaborative agreement with another health provider in order for the NP to provide patient care, or it limits the setting of one or more elements of NP practice.

Restricted Practice: State practice and licensure laws restrict the ability of NPs to engage in at least one element of NP practice. State law requires career-long supervision, delegation or team management by another health provider in order for the NP to provide patient care.

Source: State Nurse State Practice Acts and Administration Rules, 2017

©American Association of Nurse Practitioners, 2017

Update: 1.2021

of health care professionals the ability to restrict access to the market by another, competing group of health care professionals, thereby denying health care consumers the benefits of greater competition."[4] The American Association of Retired Persons (AARP) supports FPA, with additional recommendations to states to amend current SOP laws and regulations to allow nurses and APRNs to perform duties for which they have been educated and certified.[1-5] Additional health policy and consumer advocacy organizations support removing SOP barriers. These groups include, but are not limited to, the National Governors Association, Bipartisan Policy Center, and the Josiah Macy Foundation.[1]

THE CAMPAIGN FOR CONSENSUS

The NCSBN undertook several new efforts, including the Campaign for Consensus, designed to assist states in adopting the Consensus Model regulations regarding scope of practice for APRNs. This initiative helps states to achieve independent practice. The campaign aims to align individual state laws with the current best practices for healthcare regulations, licensure, accreditation, certification, and education (LACE), and strives to help consumers, employers, and other healthcare providers understand the correct scope of practice for NPs. Although nationally certified, APRNs' education is based on the Consensus Model (2008).[6] The Consensus Model for APRNs defines advanced practice registered nurse practice and describes emergence of new roles and population foci. Often referred to as LACE this model adopted the term "population focus" to describe the broad area of preparation for NPs. This landmark model defined titles to be used by NPs, defined emergence of new roles and specialty populations (or population foci), and presented strategies for implementation.[7]

Over the past several decades the APRN has become a highly valued and integral part of the healthcare system. APRNs include practitioners in the following areas: certified nurse anesthetists (CRNA), certified nurse midwives (CNM), clinical nurse specialists (CNS), and certified nurse practitioners (CNP). The uniqueness of these individual practitioners is that their role focuses on specialized knowledge and skills acquired through graduate-level education. These APRN roles focus on direct patient care. Within the NP role, there are the following specific population foci. Below is a list of the implementation date associated with each specific specialty.

- 2010 Adult-Gerontology Primary Care Nurse Practitioners
- 2012 Adult-Gerontology Acute Care Nurse Practitioners
- 2013 Primary Care Pediatric Nurse Practitioner
- 2013 Acute Care Pediatric Nurse Practitioner
- 2013 Neonatal Nurse Practitioner
- Family/Across the Lifespan Nurse Practitioner
- Women's Health/Gender Related Nurse Practitioner
- Psychiatric-Mental Health Nurse Practitioner

Specifically, the campaign lobbies for all states to incorporate these rules into their legislation:

1. Recognition of the title "nurse practitioner"
2. Licensure as both an RN and as an NP
3. Graduate or postgraduate education from an accredited institution
4. Board-issued certification in a medical specialty
5. Independent practice
6. Independent prescribing[8]

SCOPE-OF-PRACTICE

SOP laws are governed by individual state laws. SOP refers to the specific procedures, actions, and processes that a healthcare provider is legally permitted to do. SOP currently varies by state and is governed by the law. States are considering relaxing SOP laws for APRNs as a potential approach to improve access to care, maintain or enhance care quality, and decrease overall healthcare costs.[8] This is why NP SOP varies from state-to-state. The rules establish both the range of services APRNs may deliver and the extent to which APRNs are permitted to practice with or without physician supervision.[3] It is important to make the distinction that FPA does not expand the NP's SOP outside of their area of specialty certification.

FULL PRACTICE AUTHORITY

Oregon and Washington were the first states to offer expanded scope of practice in the 1980s; more rural states, mainly those with physician shortages, followed in the 1990s. Prior to the 2010 *Future of Nursing Report* by the IOM,[2] 13 states had FPA.

Nearly 8 years later, 16 more states, the District of Columbia, and 2 US territories have gained FPA (Table 12-1). In some states, FPA is granted upon successful completion of the national certification examination (Table 12-2). Fifteen states (Table 12-3) currently require varying transition to practice time frames prior to receiving FPA. As of this writing, 16 states are listed as reduced or restricted practice. All 50 states and the District of Columbia as well as 2 US territories now have prescriptive authority. However, there remain limits on prescribing of specific classes of medications.

The major challenges facing FPA remain as (1) requirements for oversight by medical rather than nursing boards, (2) clinical oversight by or collaboration with physicians, and (3) restrictions on APRNs' provisions of a range of services, including hospital admitting privileges and insurance reimbursement.[9]

TABLE 12-1

Chronology of Full Practice Authority

1980s—IOM report (13 states)	After IOM report in 2010 (16 states) + DC and 2 US territories
Idaho (1970s)	Vermont (2011)
Alaska (1984)	North Dakota
New Hampshire	Rhode Island
Oregon	Massachusetts (2013)
Wyoming	Utah
Washington	Nevada (2013)
Iowa	Connecticut (2014)
Montana	Minnesota (2014)
New Mexico	Delaware (2016)
Arkansas (1995)	Maryland (2015)
Maine (1995)	New York (2015)
Hawaii (2009)	Nebraska (2015)
Colorado (2010)	West Virginia (2016) FPA only if not prescribing
	Arizona (2016)
	District of Columbia (2017)
	South Dakota (2017)
	Guam and NMI (2018)
	Virginia (2019)

RATIONALE FOR AUTONOMY

The Patient Protection and Affordable Care Act (2010) expanded healthcare coverage for millions of Americans and further increased the demand for primary care physicians.[10]

TABLE 12-2

Upon Initial Licensure (17 + DC)

Alaska	New Hampshire
District of Columbia	Rhode Island
Hawaii	Utah
Idaho	Arizona
Iowa	Arkansas
Montana	Massachusetts
New Mexico	
North Dakota	
Oregon	
Wyoming	
Washington	

TABLE 12-3

States Requiring a Transition to Practice Period Post-Licensure Practice Period (15 States)

Illinois - 4,000 hours	Kentucky - 4 years
Maine (1995/2007) 24 months	West Virginia (2016) 2 years
Colorado (2010/2015) 1000 hours	South Dakota (2017) 1040 hours
Vermont (2011) 24 months and 2400 hours	Virginia (2019) 5 years and 9,000 hours
Nevada (2013) 2 years or 2000 hours	
Minnesota (2014) 2080 hours	
Connecticut (2014) 3 years/2000 hours	
New York (2014) 3600 hours	
Nebraska (2015) 2000 hours	
Delaware (2015) 2 years/minimum 4000 fulltime hours	
Maryland (2015) 18 months	

Petterson et al. (2012) estimated that the United States will have a shortage of just under 52,000 primary care physicians by 2025.[12] Increasing the number of NPs is one strategy to increasing the number of primary care providers.[12] Increasing the types of primary care providers improves patient access and decreases wait times to see a provider.

As early as 1981 (reconfirmed in 1986) the United States Office of Technology Assessment concluded from examination of NP care and practice patterns that NPs perform as well as physicians in all areas of primary care delivery and health outcomes.[13,14] Nurse practitioners are well positioned to impact a positive change in healthcare and develop new models of healthcare delivery. AANP has a well-documented body of literature that supports the position that NPs provide care that is safe, effective, patient-centered, timely, efficient, equitable, and evidence-based.[15]

Although NPs were initially certified and employed in primary care settings the mid-1990s saw the development of the acute care nurse practitioner (ACNP) role. This inpatient NP role was developed largely because of the human resource need due to the shortage of critical care physicians. The restrictions of resident physician practice/duty hours (as a result of changes in graduate medical education) reduced the number of care providers in the hospital setting.[15] The ACNP role was designed to help meet these coverage needs as well as to implement quality directives.[16,17] Care coordination and transitions of care are extremely important to positive patient outcomes of hospital care, for all patients, regardless of age.[7]

The American population continues to age, creating an increased need for both primary care and hospital-based NP services. While primary care NPs focus on increasing access to care and decreased wait times, ACNPs focus on decreasing lengths of stay and intervention outcomes.

FPA for NPs enables them to provide patients with direct access to the full services that NPs can provide.[18] The AANP outlines the benefits of FPA (Table 12-4).[1] One of the benefits of FPA is that it will

TABLE 12-4

Benefits of FPA

FPA benefit to patient care	Method/Rationale	Other considerations
Improved patient access	Delivers care to under-served and rural areas Allows increased service to an aging population	Addresses primary care provider workforce shortage Addresses change in Graduate Medical Education duty-hour requirements
Streamlined care delivery making more efficient	Provides direct patient access to providers Removes delays in care when dated regulations require a physician signature prior to initiation of medications or diagnostic testing	Assures timely access to care
Decreased cost	Avoids duplication of services and billing costs related to physician oversight Reduces repetition of orders, office visits, and other services	Medicare payments to NPs are at 85% of the physician fee schedule This is in alignment with many commercial payers
Protects patients' right to choose	Allows patient access to healthcare provider of their choice	Removes constraint on the practice of one health discipline in a regulating relationship with another profession

FPA, Full Practice Authority; NP, nurse practitioner.

Source: Data from AANP materials and Dillon and Gary.[20]

"free up physician time" that is currently being utilized for authorization of prescriptions and medical treatments. It is felt that patient satisfaction will also improve as patients' will experience decreased office wait times, both in scheduling of appointments (improving access to care) as well as during the actual office visit.

BARRIERS TO FULL PRACTICE AUTHORITY

Physician Barriers

Multiple barriers to FPA continue to exist. Physicians do not feel that NPs are educationally prepared and will create a two-class system of healthcare, one that is physician-led and another that is led by "less-qualified health professionals."[19] The American Academy of Family Physicians (AAFP) issued their report (2012) taking issue with NPs and FPA. They acknowledged the valuable role played by advanced practitioners in the healthcare team, but dually noted that NPs "cannot fulfill the need for a fully trained physician."[19] The report contained multiple errors related to the NPs educational preparation and ability to arrive at an initial diagnosis. The report was quickly countered by Dr. Bobbie Berkowitz, Dean of the Columbia School of Nursing in New York City, for its multiple flaws and lack of data to support its statements.[20] She stated that the report from the AAFP was contrary to the recommendations from the IOM and the NCSBN as well as "being contrary to the requirements set forth by the National Committee for Quality Assurance (NCQA) and The Joint Commission.[21] She also acknowledged that despite 40 years of evidence to the contrary, the AAFP report made the misleading statement that NPs misdiagnose, miss obvious and potentially life-threatening problems, or make prescribing errors.[21]

Insurance Payer Barriers

Barriers from the insurance payer market also face NPs in their desire to achieve FPA. There are still commercial insurance carriers that do not recognize NPs as primary care providers on their panels. Frequently, payer policies are linked to state practice regulations and licensure.[22] Reimbursement by commercial health insurance carriers for NP services may also be fixed at 80% to 85% of the standard physician fee reimbursement for delivery of the same service. Updating scope of practice legislation to be in alignment with FPA will assist in lobbying for changes in current insurance reimbursement.

Federal and State Barriers

The Social Security Act, which governs Medicare and Medicaid, was written in 1965.[23,25] These documents were developed in the very early years of NP role implementation. Although there have been revisions made in the documents since that time, there are still portions that give only permission to physicians to provide care. The act still states that a physician must direct the care of hospitalized patients.[25] The Centers for Medicare and Medicaid Services (CMS) require hospitalized Medicare patients to be "under the care of a doctor of medicine or osteopathy" (481.12).[24] The act further states that this certification is required for hospital inpatient coverage and payment under Medicare Part A and may be signed only by one of the following: (1) a physician who is a doctor of medicine or osteopathy, (2) a dentist in the circumstances specified in 42 CFR 424.13 (d), or (3) a doctor of podiatric medicine if his or her certification is consistent with the functions he or she is authorized to perform under state law.[24] These acts are incorporated into hospital medical staff bylaws and pose as additional barriers to NP practice.

In addition to updating Federal legislation, state nursing licensure laws also need to be updated to meet current practice and population healthcare needs.[18] Part of this process is removing requirements for collaborative practice with physician providers. This legislation would enable patients to benefit from NP services in a variety of settings including hospitals, nursing homes, home healthcare, and hospice environments.

LOCAL BARRIERS

In addition to the aforementioned barriers to practice, health-care system medical staff bylaws may further restrict APRN practice. Impacting change in all of these areas is essential for APRN's to be able to practice at their full level of their licensure and certification.

SUMMARY

FPA for NPs has had a long and challenging history. The challenge will continue until all states receive FPA. This history continues to be written today as many states are still practicing under a reduced or restrictive practice model. NPs lobbying at the state and national levels are needed to help advance practice and update outdated legislation. The evidence is supportive that NPs provide care that is cost-effective, with either no difference between MD and NP providers or evidence of a reduction in morbidity and mortality under NP care.[26–29] NPs have a professional duty to educate stakeholders such as the public and legislators as to the existing evidence supporting the aforementioned axioms. This action would enable NPs to implement the IOM recommendations that state, "The current conflicts between what APRNs can do based on their education and training and what they may do according to state and federal regulations must be resolved so that they are better able to provide seamless, affordable and quality care."[2] NP advocacy is one way to become involved in changing scope of practice and moving the needle toward FPA for all.

References

1. American Academy of Nurse Practitioners. *Issues At-A-Glance: Full Practice Authority.* http://www/aanp.org. Updated 2013. Accessed September 20, 2020.

2. Institute of Medicine. (2010). *The Future of Nursing: Leading Change, Advancing Health.* Washington, DC: National Academies Press. http://www.iom.edu.Reports/2010/The-Future-of-Nursing-Leading-Change-Advancing-Health.aspx. Accessed September 20, 2020.

3. American Nurses Association (ANA). (2011). *ANA, CMA, and OA Activities Reflected in the IOM Recommendations.* http://www.nursingworld.org/ANA-Activities-IOM-Report. Accessed September 20, 2020.

4. Gilman, D.J. & Koslov, T.I. (2014, March). Federal Trade Commissions. *Policy Perspectives: Competition and the Regulation of Advance Practice Nurses.* Washington, DC: Federal Trade Commission. http://www.ftc.gov/reports/policy-perspectives-competition-regulation-advanced-practice-nurses. Accessed September 20, 2020.

5. Brassard, A. & Smolenk, M. (2012). *Removing Barriers to Advance Practice Registered Nurse Care: Hospital Privileges* (pp. 1–12). Washington, DC: AARP Public Policy Institute.

6. *Consensus Model for APRN Regulation: Licensure, Accreditation, Certification & Education.* (2008, July 7). APRN Joint Dialogue Group. Retrieved from APRN Consensus Model. www.nursingworld.org/consensusmodel. Accessed September 20, 2020.

7. American Association of Colleges of Nursing. www.aacnnursing.org. Accessed September 20, 2020.

8. DeCapua, M. Scope of Practice vs Independent Practice—What's the Difference. https://www.bartonassociates.com/blg/np-scope-of-practice-vs-independent-practice-whats-the-difference/. Accessed September 20, 2020.

9. Martsolf, G.R., Auerbach, D.I., & Arifkhanova, A. The Impact of Full Practice Authority for Nurse Practitioners and Other Advanced Practice Registered Nurses in Ohio. https://www.rand.org/t/rr848. Accessed September 20, 2020.

10. *Assessing Progress on the Institute of Medicine Report The Future of Nursing.* The National Academies Press. http://nap.edu/21838. Accessed June 8, 2018.

11. US Department of Health and Human Services. The Patient Protection and Affordable Care Act (2010).

12. Petterson, S.M., Winston, R.L., Phillips, R.L., Rabin, D.L., Meyers, D.S., & Bazemore, A.W. (2012, November–December). Projecting U.S. Primary Care Physician Workforce Needs: 2010–2025. *Annals of Family Medicine,* 10 (6), 503–509.

13. Weinburg, M.P. (2014). *Full Practice Authority for Nurse Practitioners Increases Access and Controls Cost* (pp. 1–20). San Francisco, CA: Bay Area Council Economic Institute.

14. US Congress, Office of Technology Assessment. (1981). *The Cost Effectiveness of Nurse Practitioners.* Washington, DC: US Government Printing Office.

15. US Congress, Office of Technology Assessment. (1986). *Nurse Practitioners, Physician Assistants, and Certified Nurse Midwives. A Policy Analysis.*

Washington, DC: US Government Printing Office. Library of Congress Card No. 85-600596.

16. American Association of Nurse Practitioners. Quality of Nurse Practitioner Practice. http://www.aanp.org. Updated 2013. Accessed September 20, 2020.

17. Nasca, T.J., Day, S.H., & Amis, E.S. Jr; ACGME Duty Hour Task Force. (2010). The New Recommendations on Duty Hours from the ACGME Task Force. *New England Journal of Medicine,* 363 (2) e3.

18. Kapu, A.N., Kleinpell, R.M., & Pilon, B. (2014). Quality and Financial Impact of Adding Nurse Practitioners to Inpatient Care Teams. *The Journal of Nursing Administration,* 44 (2) 87–96.

19. Burns, S. & Earven, S. (2002). Improving Outcomes for Mechanically Ventilated Medical Intensive Care Unit Patients Using Advanced Practice Nurses: A 6-Year Experience. *Critical Care Nursing Clinics of North America,* 14 231–243.

20. Dillon D. & Gary, F. (2017). Full Practice Authority for Nurse Practitioners. *Nursing Administration Quarterly,* 41 (1) 86–93.

21. Goertz, R. (2012). Independent Practice Authority for Nurse Practitioners Could Splinter Care, Undermine Patient-Centered Medical Home. *Annals of Family Medicine,* 10 (6) 572–573.

22. American Association of Nurse Practitioners. Press Releases & Announcements. AANP Responds to American Academy of Family Physicians Report. http://www.Aanp.org/press-releases/1082. Published 2012. Accessed September 20, 2020.

23. Mills, C. Why NPs Need Full Practice and Prescriptive Authority. *Nurse Practitioner World News,* May–June 2009.

24. Hain, D., Fleck, L.M. (2014). Barriers to NP Practice that Impact Healthcare Redesign. *The Online Journal of Issues in Nursing,* 19 (2) 2.

25. The Social Security Act, 42 USCS 1395 €(4). http://www.gpo.gov/fdsys/pkg/USCODE:2011-title42/html/USCOD. Accessed September 20, 2020.

26. Centers for Medicare and Medicaid Services. Hospital Inpatient Admission Order and Certification. http://www.CMS.gov. Accessed September 20, 2020.

27. Gershengorn, H.B., Wunish, H., & Wahab, R. (2011). Impact of Non-Physician Staffing on Outcomes in a Medical ICU. *Chest,* 139 (6) 1347–1353.

28. Skinner, H.S.J., Redfearn, S., Jutley, R., Mitchell, I., & Richens, D. (2013). Advanced Care Nurse Practitioners Can Safely Provide Sole Resident Cover for Levels Three Patients: Impact on Outcomes, Cost and Work Patterns in a Cardiac Surgery Programme. *European Journal of Cardio Thoracic Surgery,* 43 (1) 19–22.

29. Scherr, K., Wilson, D.M., Wagner, J., & Haughianm, M. (2012). Evaluating a New Rapid Response Team: NP Led-versus Intensivist-Led Comparisons. *AACN Advanced Critical Care,* 23 (1) 32–42.

INDEX

Pages with *f* indicate figures and pages with *t* indicate tables.

C